INSIDE MANAGED CARE

Family Therapy in a
Changing Environment

INSIDE MANAGED CARE

Family Therapy in a
Changing Environment

Jodi Aronson, Ph.D., LMFT

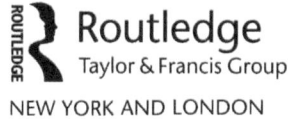

Routledge
Taylor & Francis Group

NEW YORK AND LONDON

The publisher would like to thank William A. Griffin, Ph.D.,
Associate Professor and Director, Marriage and Family Therapy
Program, Arizona State University, for his efforts on behalf of this
book.

First published 1996 by Brunner/Mazel, Inc.

This edition published 2014 by Routledge
711 Third Avenue, New York, NY 10017, USA
27 Church Road, Hove East Sussex, BN3 2FA

Routledge is an imprint of the Taylor & Francis Group, an informa business

Library of Congress Cataloging-in-Publication Data

Aronson, Jodi.
    Inside managed care: family therapy in a changing environment /
by Jodi Aronson.
        p.   cm.
    Includes bibliographical references and index.
    ISBN 0-87630-818-3 (pbk.)
    1. Family psychotherapy.   2. Managed care plans (Medical care)
I. Title.
RC488.5.A76   1996
616.89'156–dc20   96-28522
                                                           CIP

About the Author

Jodi Aronson holds a doctorate degree in family therapy and is a licensed marriage and family therapist in the state of Florida. She is a member of the American Association for Marriage and Family Therapists (AAMFT), as well as an AAMFT Approved Supervisor. Dr. Aronson is the Central Regional Care Center Director of MCC Behavioral Care, Inc., which is a wholly owned subsidiary of CIGNA Health Care. In addition to working in the managed care market for the past four years, she has been an adjunct professor at Nova Southeastern University in Ft. Lauderdale, Florida.

This book is dedicated to my family
who has been supportive and loving with no limit.

Contents

Foreword

The revolution is under way. Not since the days of Thomas Sazaz and his challenges to the state of mental health thinking in the United States, and not since the development of community mental health and the deinstitutionalization of psychiatric patients under the administration of John F. Kennedy, has this country seen such radical and sweeping changes in the area of mental health care. In spite of the noble goals of the Clinton Administration, and particularly the efforts by Hillary Rodham Clinton, Congress once again refused to be proactive in promoting health care reform. However, the mental health industry is rapidly reinventing itself and the evolutionary process will not be stopped.

Managed care companies have played, and are playing a critical role in the process of change that is occurring. I remember during the early 1970s, when in graduate school at the University of Louisville, I first heard of HMO services from a professor of mine. He and his family had been covered under an HMO when they lived in California, and he complained of not being able to secure such services in Kentucky. He spoke highly of the HMO concept and of the services that he and his family had received. Recent communications from the mental health industry often lack that type of affirmation and tend to focus on the negative issues and complaints, such as loss of autonomy and loss of control. Unfortunately, often missing from that discourse have been the voices of those professionals who are thriving and have been able to work collaboratively with managed care. Many of us have been glad to see positive value placed on what I have often described as "sensible psychotherapy." Many of us are pleased to struggle with the dichotomy of our therapy's being art and science. For us, it is not an either/or proposition, but a both/and proposition.

What family therapists need to negotiate the complex terrain of managed care is a good road map and clinical guide. Dr. Aronson has provided us with just that in this book. The content is pragmatic and will serve as an excellent primer to begin to understand the complex world of managed care. The clinical case examples are rich and demonstrate effectiveness and positive outcome. The book incorporates the voices of therapists who are partners in a creative endeavor to provide high quality services to a wide range of clients. The case examples also provide a clear picture of how various clinical approaches can be utilized in such a managed care context and how effective outcome is, more often than not, multidisciplinary and team based.

Whether or not one is a proponent of managed care, there can be no doubt that the revolution/evolution will continue. This book will be helpful to those who wish to be a constructive part of that change. In 1989, I gave a series of lectures to mental health professionals in Norway and in Germany regarding the need to deconstruct the mental health industry in the United States. Now the time has come to construct the one that will carry us into the 21st century.

Tom Russell, LCSW, LMFT
Regional Clinical Director
Central Region
MCC Behavioral Care, Inc.

Acknowledgments

I would like to extend a special note of gratitude to all therapists and case managers who shared their stories with me. In addition, I would like to thank Tom Russell, Betty Davis, and Paul Maione for their time and thoughtful feedback as this book matured.

Introduction

Over the past few years, therapists have been introduced to and educated in managed mental health care (Poynter, 1994). In this time, therapists have come to understand that the only true stability in managed care is the fact that it is ever changing. However, even in this ever-changing environment, there are a number of themes that remain consistent. If there are themes that remain constant, why don't therapists know them? Because they have not been privy to an insider's look at managed mental health care. Until now.

This book takes you inside managed care to show both how the MCOs work and the importance of the family therapist's clear documentation of sound clinical judgments. In addition, this book looks at brief systemic therapies and how they fit into a managed market.

One core theme that remains constant is the fact that Managed Care Organizations (MCOs) maintain the goal of trying to deliver quality care in the least intrusive manner possible while controlling costs for all partners. For this reason, as well as many others that will be discussed in this book, family therapists have a natural marriage with MCOs. Believing in and maintaining a systemic perspective means that clients' problems can be more easily addressed and solved. By working from the perspective that the problem lies in the context and not in the individual (Bateson, Jackson, Haley, & Weakland, 1956), the brief systemic therapist is aligned to find symptom relief in a short time. This is an attractive prospect to employer groups as they battle rising costs in health care. In addition, MCOs are faced with the struggle of providing quality care within limited benefit packages.

Family therapists are comfortable in dealing with multiple customers. For example, it is very rare that every member of a family wants the same outcome from therapy. The family therapist has mastered the skill of maintaining maneuverability. This skill is one highly valued by MCOs as the MCO needs to maintain its maneuverability among numerous customers who present with a variety of needs. The MCO is the liaison between the employer and the employee as it relates to insurance benefits. For example, the MCO will offer the employer an array of benefit programs to implement with the employee group. The employer will choose the benefit package based on need, financial analysis, and quality analysis. Once the employer decides on the programs to offer the employees, the employees choose from a limited menu. Once the employees enroll in the benefit program, the MCO is responsible for managing the benefits in ways that keep employees healthy so that they remain productive at work.

The idea commonly expressed by therapists that MCOs are intrusive and force the therapist to lose his/her autonomy need not be the case if the therapist understands the inner workings of MCOs. In addition, family therapists are nicely situated to gain more of the market share as they learn how to better sell their wares to the MCOs. In the past, and in some instances in the present, family therapists have not been granted entrée to provider panels. This is a loss to the MCOs, which need to be further educated as to the true meaning of "family therapy," which is better described as "systems therapy." An example: when parents call into the MCO to have services arranged for their 5-year-old child. If the MCO does not believe in a systemic approach to treatment, an assessment with a child psychologist will more than likely be set up for the child. This strengthens the parent's belief that the child has pathologies, and the child will be dropped off at weekly therapy sessions. The therapist may spend a few moments with the parents at the end of each session to summarize the session.

However, when MCOs fully understand the value of systemic family treatment, the family therapist will be more valued as a treatment provider who can be more clinically efficacious and more cost-effective for such a case. The family therapist would likely see the family as an entity and evaluate what is defined as the problem in the context that the problem occurs. As MCOs have increasingly recognized this value, family therapists are finding themselves on MCO panels in greater numbers.

The author found herself working for an MCO by mistake. Once believing that MCOs did not make room for family therapists on the panels or on staff at the organization, this writer was very surprised when a job interview at a group practice turned into a job providing clinical care for an MCO. Once introduced to the inside workings of an MCO, it became apparent that there was a budding relationship between marriage and family therapists and MCOs. This book provides an insider's view of the world of MCOs as it pertains to family therapists, as well as to any therapist who embraces the systems perspective.

1

Here's What Everyone Needs to Know

Once therapists* understand the language that the managed care company uses, they will be better prepared to work with the case managers who will review their treatment. This chapter begins by looking at various benefit programs and how a given program may affect the clinical treatment plan. For example, a basic Health Maintenance Organization (HMO) may have a yearly limit of only 20 outpatient sessions. This limit would cover the care by the therapist and any psychiatric sessions that may be needed as well. By looking at different benefit programs, therapists will begin to understand the importance of working from a systemic, brief model of therapy.

---

*Because many therapists are not family therapists but do work in a brief systemic fashion, the word "therapist" or "provider" will be used synonymously with "family therapist" throughout this book.

So often, the key to surviving in a system is to understand the language of the context. This correlation could not be more clear than in the world of therapy where the key to successful therapy is to meet the client* where the client is (Rosen, 1982; de Shazer, 1985). However, to be a successful therapist means more than simply to provide good therapy. In order to be a successful therapist, the practitioner needs also to understand the language of doing business—the business of doing therapy. One of the largest segments in the world of therapy today is managed care (Poynter, 1994). Many practitioners hear the term "managed care" and become anxious, but it does not need to be this way. Learn the language, learn the players, learn how to play. This process is isomorphic to the process of therapy.

The first step to understanding the business of therapy is to understand the various benefit programs in which a client may be enrolled. The following scenarios give pragmatic examples of the various types of insurance programs.

Jonathan is enrolled in an HMO. The HMO has a network of providers who are credentialed. This means that the HMO has: verified the provider's education; verified the provider's liability insurance; established a written contract with the provider; interviewed the provider to get a clear understanding of the provider's specialties; and conducted a site visit to assure that the provider has an acceptable, handicapped-accessible, and secure office. The client may only have benefit coverage if a contracted provider is utilized. Therefore, Jonathan must contact the MCO to receive a referral to a contracted provider when he wants to utilize his benefits, as all of his care must be precertified.

Jonathan has 20 outpatient sessions in a contracted year and each session has a copayment of $10. When Jonathan goes to see a therapist, he is financially responsible for only

---

*The word "client" will be used synonymously with "family client."

his copayment. The therapist, who is under contract, must make sure that all the subsequent care is precertified by following the guidelines of the particular MCO. It is usual and customary that if a provider does not follow the procedures for obtaining ongoing (concurrent) authorizations, the provider shall hold the client financially harmless. In addition, the care requested by the provider will be reviewed by the MCO case managers to determine if the services are medically necessary. Only care that is medically necessary will be authorized.

Matthew is enrolled in a Preferred Provider Organization (PPO). The PPO has a network of providers with whom the MCO has contracted in order to get guaranteed reduced prices. Matthew was supplied with a directory of providers when he enrolled in the program. When Matthew wants to use the services, he only needs to call one of the providers in the directory. As the provider selection is different from that of the HMO, so is the financial arrangement of the PPO.

Matthew has an outpatient limit of $1,500 per calendar year after he meets a $300 deductible. His provider has a contracted rate and Matthew is responsible for a specified coinsurance. In Matthew's case, his coinsurance is 10% of the contracted rate. Matthew's care will not be managed clinically or financially. It is Matthew's responsibility to keep track of the amount of money accumulated. In addition to Matthew's in-network benefits, his PPO program also includes out-of-network benefits. If Matthew should choose to see a provider who is not on his preferred list, he would be responsible for a 30% coinsurance. There most likely would not be discounted rates for an out-of-network provider and, therefore, the 30% is of billable charges.

Sylvia's employer has purchased an Employee Assistance Program (EAP). The EAP is a prepaid service that allows Sylvia to get a free assessment and referral. This is particularly helpful when Sylvia knows she has a problem but is not sure what kind of services she needs. The services generally covered by an EAP are assessment and referral, legal counseling, and financial counseling, as well as a referral source to community-based services. This benefit is available to all the members of Sylvia's household even if they are not covered by her major medical insurance. The EAP is set up to be an assessment program so there are usually no barriers to access.

Sylvia can easily access this benefit by calling the Employee Assistance Program and explaining her situation. The intake specialist will either provide Sylvia with the information requested or refer Sylvia to an EAP-contracted provider for an assessment. When Sylvia goes to the EAP provider, she has no financial responsibility; the EAP provider will be reimbursed by the EAP program based on the contracted rate. The EAP provider will make a referral and help Sylvia get connected to the appropriate services. In addition, the EAP will perform a follow-up to make sure that Sylvia is comfortable with the referrals provided. If she is not, new referrals will be offered.

Jennifer has insurance coverage under an indemnity/managed indemnity plan. This is a traditional insurance program with a deductible and an 80/20 split. The only portion of her care that the insurance company reserves the right to manage would be surgical or inpatient services. This is done to make sure that the care is medically necessary. Whenever Jennifer needs services, she goes to any licensed professional she selects. She is financially responsible for meeting her $500 deductible, after which she will be responsible for paying 20% of the professional's fees. Some professionals accept assignment, whereas others expect payment in full and the insurance reimbursement is then forwarded to the client.

Under an indemnity or managed indemnity, any licensed professional can accept third party payment. Under the PPO, third party payment will be available to providers who have a contract for reduced fees. Providers usually have the most questions about becoming credentialed for a HMO/MCO.

There are many reasons for an MCO's wanting to credential its providers. These reasons include, but are not limited to, assuring quality of service, establishing/documenting quality of care, defining quality, and meeting specifications of credentialing bodies. Although providers are often put off by the need to supply a large amount of information when becoming credentialed, they must be prepared to do so.

Credentialing requirements often include information regarding quality care reviews. Quality care reviews are focused on how therapy is done and the effectiveness of such therapy. Therapists who are trying to become MCO panel members may run such studies themselves. There is much literature on outcome studies (Giles, 1993), but the point is that the study that is designed must not be too cumbersome. Simple follow-up studies may provide all the information needed to show that the therapy was effective. Therapists should get permission from their clients to contact them by telephone 90 days after therapy is completed. A simple questionnaire can be formulated to query the client about his/her impressions of achieved goals and the process of therapy.

Utilization review based on average length of treatment by diagnosis may be another tool for credentialing. An MCO may ask you what your average length of treatment is. The answer to this question can often be deceiving, especially if you have a high level of chronicity in your client load. Therefore, it behooves therapists to gather these numbers ahead of time and break the response down by diagnosis. For instance, the therapist should have a lower average number of sessions for adjustment disorders and V-Codes than for major depressive episodes.

MCOs are very interested in the voices of their members. Therefore, member satisfaction surveys are usually part of the credentialing/recredentialing process.

Therapists can easily produce and administer their own satisfaction survey to show how their services are perceived. A simple and brief Likart Scale questionnaire can be filled out by clients as they sit in the waiting room. Questions regarding office surroundings, helpfulness of support staff, therapists' understanding of the problem, and confidence in the therapist will indicate to MCOs how your clients perceive you and your services. And therapists should not feel obligated to filter out responses that are not overly favorable, as it is expected that clients do not always find a good fit with provided services.

In addition, on-site visits with structured review of medical records may be conducted. During the site visit, the MCO will make sure that the office surroundings are adequate, that the office is handicapped accessible, that the therapeutic space is presentable, and that the clinical charts are kept in a secured place. Questions that might be asked on the site visit may revolve around clinical specialties. The application and site visit provide opportunities to show that you, the family therapist, are a natural match with the MCO. This is your opportunity to educate the MCO representative about how your ability to do family therapy allows you to help find solutions that incorporate all parties who may be involved with the problem. This is also a good time to explain the benefits of brief systemic therapy.

Some of the other information that the MCO will look for is administrative in nature. The MCO may gather information about your managed care experience and may ask you to produce a list of all the MCOs with which you are currently connected. In addition, the MCO will gather information regarding the provider's current license, work history, liability claims history, legal history, and malpractice insurance, as well as get a statement attesting to good physical and mental health. All of these are ways for the MCO to make sure that therapists are who they say they are. The MCO will verify the information and materials that are provided. Although this may all seem a nuisance, it protects clients as much as it does MCOs. In addition, such vigilance protects therapists since the MCO evaluates whether a given therapist is a good match for their services. If it turns out that the therapist and the MCO are not compatible, the process will have saved the therapist a lot of time and much energy trying to fit in.

Just as speaking the language of your client is necessary, when approaching an MCO you need to speak its language—business. You want to explain to the MCO that family therapy is not only time-effective, it is cost-effective in that the goals of systemic family therapy include helping the client/client family find solutions to problems that are applicable across many life problems. This may mean fewer representations to therapy down the road. And, should the client represent, the likelihood is that it will probably be more for a mental health check (a reintroduction to the learned solutions) than long-term treatment. It is also important to present this in a realistic light. For example, solution-oriented approaches may not work with all clients; they work effectively with approximately 70% of all presentations (O'Hanlon & Weiner-Davis, 1989). Finally, it is important to indicate how your method of working can help with more severe presentations and can help to deescalate high-risk situations.

For example, if the MCO had a client who suffered from psychotic episodes, you would want to explain how you would bring the family into session to better educate them about the problem, and to enlist their help in recognizing the signs of when the identified client is starting to become disoriented. You would also want to describe how the client would be educated on how to use the family as a support system or be assisted in developing natural support systems in the absence of traditional families. Besides the basic clinical functions, you need to clarify for the MCO how your clinical skills translate naturally into case coordination and case management (discussed in Chapter 6).

2

The Scaffolding

This chapter focuses on the identifying information for each client/family that is necessary to obtain in order to retain authorization from the MCO. This easy how-to approach will help therapists remain organized both for their own private practice and for MCO requirements. In addition, sample forms are provided to help therapists understand the administrative world of managed care.

After the client calls the MCO and is given a referral to the provider, the client will call the provider to make the first appointment. Some MCOs will forward the intake information to the provider in detail, others will not. If the information is not sent, the provider can gather the demographic intake briefly.

The provider will want to get the name, address, home and work phone numbers, type of insurance coverage, date of birth and gender of the registered client, and the name of the group, employer, and the Social Security number of the insured. The MCO should have obtained a brief description of the problem, history of treatment, name of the family physician, and any substance abuse history during the telephonic intake process. The MCO would have gathered this information in order to make an appropriate referral. The provider may want to gather this information in order to determine the scheduling need of the client. If the case is urgent, then the provider will need to schedule the appointment quickly (e.g., within 48 hours). This type of responsiveness is critical to both the client and the MCO.

DEVELOP GOOD DOCUMENTATION

The most significant aspect of the provider's case file is clear and precise documentation. This starts with a good understanding of why the client is coming to therapy. In addition, such documentation helps set up the boundaries for treatment. Probably the most important document a therapist could have on file is the therapeutic treatment plan. This treatment plan includes the demographic and clinical information that is required by law to be in each clinical file (e.g., Florida Law 495.54). An organized treatment plan will help the MCO case managers to follow your treatment.

The demographic information found on a treatment plan may include, but is not restricted to, the client/family name, the client's address, the client's date of birth, the client's phone number, the insurance subscriber's name and Social Security number, and the subscriber's employer. This information helps the MCO to identify the client's records and to verify the subscriber's eligibility for benefits. Some MCOs may provide a form for supplying this information. Therapists should ask the case manager which is preferred. One shortcut may be for the provider to gather copies of all treatment plan forms from all of the MCOs with which the therapist is contracted (remember to keep an original on file so you can always have a supply available).

Map out the breadth of information requested from these companies and collect these data on each client whether a particular MCO is asking for the data or not.

For example, MCO "X" may ask for employer name and address, whereas MCO "Y" doesn't want that information but asks for the Social Security numbers of the client and subscriber. If therapists simply get into the habit of gathering the most comprehensive of demographic information, they will be better prepared for all MCOs and will not need to remember different rules for various companies.

Each state outlines under its mental health laws information that is mandated to be part of a mental health file. The majority of states require that the mental health professional inquire about and document a client's medical history. Besides satisfying the needs of the mental health law, such medical background provides therapists with pertinent information, which may be needed when managing the care of the client. Therapists can incorporate this information into general information forms, which allows for the building of a client data file without intruding on the therapy. This information should include a history of mental health treatments, surgeries, and allergies, and a list of current medications. It is also recommended that therapists obtain a release from the client to communicate with the client's primary care physician.

Aside from the foregoing, the clinical information found on a treatment plan would include a brief description of the presenting problem, the DSM-IV diagnosis, the current symptoms in behavioral terms, current medications if applicable, current dosages of the medications, and any pathological use of alcohol, psychoactive substances, and/or illicit drugs. The treatment plan should also include the goals of treatment (in behavioral terms), psychosocial information, and mental status examination information. Other important points might be the criteria for termination of the current phase of treatment and the estimated duration of treatment.

Exhibit 2.1 is an example of what a treatment plan form might look like.

Treatment Plan

Date of Assessment _____

Name _____ Social Security Number _____

Subscriber's Name and Social Security Number
_____

Presenting Problem:
_____
_____

Psychosocial:

Age ____ Race ____ Marital Status _____ # of Children ____

Other: _____
_____
_____

Mental Status:
_____
_____
_____

Diagnosis:

Axis I _____   Axis II _____   Axis III _____

        Axis IV _____   Axis V _____

Treatment Plan:

Goals: _____
_____
_____
_____

Action Plan:

CPT Code _____   Frequency _____

Estimated length of treatment _____

Other suggestions _____
_____

_____   _____
Signature and Credentials   Date

Exhibit 2.1. Sample treatment plan form.

Although the form may be self-explanatory, filling it out "correctly" can often be confusing. Formalizing treatment goals that MCO case managers can understand may become complicated. In order to clarify the process, the following MCO case was chosen to exemplify how case information is translated for the treatment form.

Mary is a 29-year-old woman. She has been married for four years and has a one-year-old daughter. She has never been in treatment before. She called to access her mental health benefits because she has been feeling upset lately. She is having trouble sleeping, eating, and staying focused at work. She is a school teacher. Mary stated that she and her husband have been fighting a lot recently over the new day care arrangements at the paternal grandparents' home. Mary's father-in-law has a long standing alcohol problem, but it had never caused a problem until recently when he passed out while he was alone with his granddaughter. Mary's in-laws are now not speaking to her.

The presenting problem described is the story that Mary presented to the therapist during the first session. There are a number of ways to gather the demographic information. Some therapists use a portion of the first session to get therapy business out of the way. This may include gathering demographic information, explaining cancellation policy, explaining emergency reporting, setting a fee schedule, and/or explaining insurance coverage. Other therapists prefer to gather the demographic information through a questionnaire prior to seeing the client. This leaves the first session purely for clinical exploration. Exhibit 2.2 is a completed treatment plan for Mary's case.

Mary and her husband attended five sessions. They were both committed to making changes in order to improve their relationship. They both agreed to find different day care, even though Jonathan would have to get a second, part-time job in order to pay for it. They both agreed that Jonathan's parents' home was too unstable an environment for their daughter.

Treatment Plan

Date of Assessment *May 12, 1996*

Name *Mary Smith*   Social Security Number *000-00-000*

Subscriber's Name and Social Security Number
Jonathan Smith 000-000-000

Presenting Problem:

Mary presents for therapy because she is having child-care problems, marital problems, extended family problems, and depressive symptoms.

Psychosocial:

Age *29*   Race *W*   Marital Status *Married*   # of Children *1*

Other: *Father-in-law drank while child was in his care. Husband not understanding of Mary's concerns. Stress of situation impacting work and marital relationship.*

Mental Status:

Client is coherent and oriented times three. Depressed mood and affect restricted to said mood. No meds. No alcohol/drug use. No suicidal or homicidal ideation.

Diagnosis:

Axis I *309.00*   Axis II *none*   Axis III *none*

         Axis IV *V61.10*   Axis V *85/85*

Treatment Plan:

Goals: *Client to find stable day care outside of family; improve communication between wife and husband(decrease fighting over in-laws); help couple to define common goals in terms of extended family; decrease depressive symptoms in Mary.*

Action Plan:

CPT Code *90847*   Frequency *every other week*

Estimated length of treatment *11*

Other suggestions *psychiatric consult if depressive symptoms do not subside in one month.*

XXXXXXXXXXXXXX, Ph.D., LMFT   *5-29-96*

Signature and Credentials   Date

Exhibit 2.2. Sample of completed treatment plan form.

Mary wanted Jonathan to confront his parents to show them that he supported her. Jonathan felt that this would only fall on deaf ears and that deciding on new day-care arrangements should show Mary that he supported her. Although Mary's depressive symptoms subsided, she could not get over the anger she felt toward Jonathan's parents.

The therapist felt that it was important to continue the work with Jonathan and Mary since they had unresolved goals for improving their communication and making mutual decisions on how to deal with extended family. The therapist helped the couple to understand that the problem was not going to go away over night since you cannot get others to change if they are unwilling to do so. They agreed to be patient and to consider the option of bringing the extended-family members into session.

The therapist needed to give the MCO a treatment update as he was only authorized for six sessions. The treatment update is the way to communicate justification for continued authorization with the MCOs. The treatment update needs to include any changes in client/family status that show progress or regression. In addition, therapists need to document the progress made toward each goal set in the initial treatment plan. Any current medications or any medication changes since the last review should be included. Finally, the update should also include the estimated duration of treatment so that the case manager can get a clear picture of the entire course of treatment. You will need to ask each MCO how the update review is communicated. Some MCOs may do the reviews by telephone, whereas others may want the review in writing. Just as with the treatment plan, gather treatment update forms from all the MCOs, keep them on file and organize your information to cover all possible bases. Exhibit 2.3 is an example of a treatment update form. It is followed by a completed update form (Exhibit 2.4) based on Mary and Jonathan's case.

Mary and Jonathan continued in treatment. They decided

Treatment Update

Date of Assessment _____

Name _____ Social Security Number _____

Subscriber's Name and Social Security Number

_____

Presenting Problem:

_____
_____
_____

Diagnosis:

Axis I _____   Axis II _____   Axis III _____

          Axis IV _____   Axis V _____

Treatment Plan:

Achieved Goals: _____

_____
_____

Unachieved Goals: _____

_____

Plan: _____

_____

Action Plan:

CPT Code _____   Frequency _____
# of sessions to termination _____

Other suggestions _____

_____

_____   _____

Signature and Credentials   Date

Exhibit 2.3. Sample of treatment update form.

Treatment Update

Date of Assessment *6-29-96*

Name *Mary Smith*   Social Security Number *000-00-0000*

Subscriber's Name and Social Security Number

Jonathan Smith 000-00-0000

Presenting Problem:

Mary presented to therapy with marital problems after her father-in-law was drunk while taking care of her daughter. Marital conflicts, depressive symptoms.

Diagnosis:

Axis I *309.00*   Axis II *none*   Axis III *none*

Axis IV *V61.10*   Axis V *85/85*

Treatment Plan:

Achieved Goals: *Couple has been able to find new child care. Depressive symptoms subsided—better concentration at work—better eating/ sleeping.*

Unachieved Goals: *Client and husband still disagree on how to handle extended family, which cause fights and anger.*

Plan: *Work with couple to find ways to resolve anger and find healthy ways to deal with extended family.*

Action Plan:

CPT Code *90847*   Frequency *every third week*

# of sessions to termination *4*

Other suggestions *If couple is agreeable, bring extended family into treatment.*

XXXXXXXXXXXXXX, Ph.D., LMFT   *6-29-96*

Signature and Credentials   Date

Exhibit 2.4. Sample of completed treatment update form.

not to bring in the extended family because they were convinced that they could not change Jonathan's parents. They were able to reframe this as needing to establish their own autonomy. Mary still had some anger toward them because, in her mind, their inability to care for her daughter properly forced Jonathan to get an extra job to pay for outside day care, and now she did not have much time alone with her husband. The couple continued to work on this, when suddenly and unexpectedly a job transfer came in for Mary. This transfer would allow Jonathan and Mary to move to a state where they could each make more money in their primary jobs, and where Mary's corporate office would provide day care.

Upon terminating with Mary and Jonathan, the provider filed a termination report with the MCO. Such termination reports should include, but are not restricted to, the reason for ending treatment, prognosis, number of sessions, number of cancellations/no shows, and closing diagnosis. As before, therapists need to query each MCO as to how the MCO wants notification of terminations. Exhibit 2.5 is a sample of a termination report, followed by a completed form (Exhibit 2.6) for Mary and Jonathan's case.

As the number of MCOs grows in the marketplace, it can become an overwhelming task to keep up with the various types of paperwork and policies. While some companies require the paperwork just shown, others asks for different paperwork, and still others do clinical reviews by telephone. Private practitioners can get lost in a flurry of procedures that can become costly if deadlines for precertification are missed. Managed care is not a different standard; it is a way to use the number of sessions wisely and cost-effectively. Since efficiency is a mark of quality, one basic rule of thumb is to pick the company with the "strictest" standards and use those parameters for all cases.

Termination Report

Name _____ Social Security Number _____

Date of Last Session _____

Total Number of Sessions:

Individual ____

Family ____

Group ____

Current Diagnosis:

Axis I _____   Axis II _____   Axis III _____

Axis IV _____   Axis V _____

Prognosis:

Poor: ____   Fair: ____   Good: ____

Is the client involved in any other care? ____

_____   _____

Signature and Credentials   Date

Exhibit 2.5. Sample of termination report form.

Termination Report

Name *Mary Smith*   Social Security Number *000-00-0000*

Date of Last Session *8-2-96*

Total Number of Sessions:

Individual ____

Family *9*

Group ____

Current Diagnosis:

Axis I *309.28*   Axis II *none*   Axis III *none*
             Axis IV *none*   Axis V *85*

Prognosis:

Poor: ____   Fair: ____   Good: ✓

Is the client involved in any other care? *no*

XXXXXXXXXXXXXX, Ph.D., LMFT   *8-3-96*
Signature and Credentials   Date

Exhibit 2.6. Sample of completed termination report form.

Organization Tips

In an effort to obtain the practitioner's view of the possible confusion that can occur when working with various MCOs, a focus group consisting of private practitioners* who are contracted with various MCOs, was organized in Fort Lauderdale, Florida, by the author. The following are some of the tips and suggestions that were gleamed from this focus group.

- Software is an important tool for keeping various items of information straight. The office staff maintains separate ledgers for each client and the ledgers are marked with the specific MCO's names. Each ledger indicates the date by which the next piece of paperwork is due. When the front office staff does the billing, they can flag the clinical file for the paperwork that the practitioner needs to fill out.

- I have come to learn all the various paperwork required by each MCO, but sometimes have difficulty remembering which case belongs to which MCO; I don't give different services to clients based on the MCO. In order to keep my files straight, I have separate file drawers for each MCO. I use the most comprehensive forms for all cases so that I don't have to do rework (using one form that serves the needs of all MCOs.) I make sure to keep an administrative form in the front of each chart that lists the authorization number, the number of sessions authorized,

*Larry Billion, Ph.D., Boca Raton; Sandra Frujita, MS, Miami; Tony King, MS, CAP, Fort Lauderdale; Barbara Kaufman, Ph.D., Boca Raton; and Ellen Sherman, Ph.D., LMFT, Boca Raton.

when the next review is due, and whether it is to be
written or by telephone.

- The office manager simply uses a colored-dot
  system. Each managed care company gets its own
  color dot and there is a cheat sheet in our front
  office that explains the policies for each managed
  care company.

- I keep a ledger sheet or a tickler system in each chart.
  It spells out the amount of the copayment. I pull
  them weekly. If a client did not show for an appointment, I place a call or send a letter. I mark the activ-
  ity on the ledger sheet. If I get no response from the
  client, I close the case. The ledger is a simple
  reminder.

- In my office we keep the different MCO cases in
  different color files. In the front office we keep a
  cheat sheet of what the different companies require.

All in all, the providers agreed that organization is what
helped them out the most. They stated that the simpler the
MCO keeps the process, the better it is for them. In addition, they stated that the MCOs they liked working with the
most were those that have a solution-oriented approach to
working with providers. They all agreed that they owned the
responsibility for obtaining follow-up authorization and that
they would not inconvenience the client with this process.

Important Points to Keep in Mind

Therapists need to stay focused on moving forward. Many
therapists can anticipate being approached by MCOs regarding shared risks, forming group practices with or without

walls, and developing clinical programs for high-acuity clients. The therapists who are open to moving into such ventures will most likely be considered preferred providers.

As MCOs vie for market shares, they are looking at ways to reduce the financial risk of doing business. Some MCOs will develop programs where financial risk is moved to a subcapitated network. This means that the MCO pays a set fee per member per month for the provider to manage the care. Other MCOs will develop programs where the MCO and the provider share risk. They might establish case rate programs, wherein the MCO pays the provider up front for an episode of care. The negotiated rate would cover all services that the therapist provides to the client.

The described programs not only shift the financial risk to the provider, they shift the quality control away from the MCO. For this reason, some MCOs may look for other options, such as finding providers in group practices, which would mean that care could be coordinated at one office. This type of arrangement allows the MCO to better access appointments for the clients. Another option for the group practice is the group practice without walls. In this setup, many providers of multidisciplinary backgrounds coordinate administrative services (i.e., intake coordination, administrative staff, on-call services), but are not all under the same roof.

The MCOs will look for clinical programs that serve clients who present for being at risk for hospitalization. Intensive outpatient programs that provide multiple group sessions and weekly individual and family sessions will be valued by MCOs. These programs can help to stabilize clients enough possibly to avoid hospitalization or they can serve as stepdown programs when a client is being discharged from a hospital stay. Therapists who can provide a program that can help to avoid hospitalization or readmission to a hospital will be considered preferred providers.

Therapists should plan for systemic programs to keep themselves well situated in the managed care market and well positioned to anticipate future trends. Family therapists are perfectly aligned to do much of this business as they are no strangers to case management. This should be emphasized as the strong point of your clinical programs.

3

Working with Employee Assistance Programs

This chapter focuses on therapists being a part of Employee Assistance Programs (EAPs). Being a provider for an EAP is a great opportunity to learn more about the world of managed care. Family therapists are best prepared to do a thorough systemic assessment to help channel individuals and families to the proper course of treatment.

Simply defined, an EAP is an assessment or brief counseling program that the employer purchases for employees and all of their household members. Employees usually contact the EAP when they need to be connected with a therapist who can help them define their concerns and find the proper treatment provider. The EAP providers need to be able to guarantee to the MCO that they will schedule the client within 48 hours of the initial client call. In addition to the appropriate access, therapists who provide care for EAP programs need to be willing to "work" to connect the client to care.

There are various EAP programs that the employer can purchase. The most common is the one- to three-session model. This program is designed to assess the client's needs and refer the client to the most appropriate treatment provider. The assessment can take up to three sessions, but the therapist is not obligated to utilize all three sessions. If the therapist assesses that the presenting problem can be addressed and solutions formulated within the three sessions, then it is more than likely all three sessions will be exhausted. However, if the therapist assesses that the client is going to require ongoing therapy, the therapist should work to get the client connected to mental health benefits as soon as possible. In some cases, the therapist may identify that the client has needs other than those therapy is designed to address; for example, financial counseling or legal advice. In these cases, the therapist will need to refer the client to the appropriate agencies for such services.

With EAP programs that run anywhere from 8 to 12 sessions, the goal is to provide brief therapy that allows clients to find solutions to their problems so that they do not have to utilize their mental health benefits. No matter what the type of EAP program, the therapist is going to need to learn to interface with the managed care program responsible for administering the client's mental health benefits.

AN EAP/MCO INTERFACE PROTOCOL

Although EAP programs come in various shapes and sizes, they all have one thing in common—an interface between the

EAP and the mental health benefits (Aronson, 1995), which, more frequently than not, are administered by an MCO.

Many EAP professionals have agreed that the interface with an MCO can be intrusive and a complicated process. This primary complaint regarding MCOs is that they often require clients to go through another assessment once they begin to use their mental health benefits. This is often an inconvenience to the client, and it discounts the quality work the EAP professional has already done. There are many ways that EAP professionals can make this process less complicated for themselves and for the client. The one single tool that produces the best results is an interface protocol between the EAP professional and MCO staff.

If EAP professionals are savvy about how an MCO operates, they will find it easy to establish an interface protocol with the MCO. Taking such an initiative will also let the employer group that buys the programs know of the EAP professional's willingness to work at making clients more comfortable with the referral process.

The first step to setting up an interface protocol is to get to know the care managers of the MCO with whom the EAP professionals will be working the most. Next, they should become familiar with the MCO's preferred providers and their practice patterns. In addition, they should explain to the case managers what the EAP assessment consists of. This will help to establish a sense of trust on both parts. The MCO staff will want assurance that the EAP professional will work with them to make a referral and not triangulate them by making a referral to a provider not on the MCO's network.

The EAP professional will need to investigate what the MCO's intake procedure is and obtain the client's permission to provide the intake information to the MCO to help facilitate the referral process. One of the most important things EAP professionals can do is to emphasize their willingness to establish working relationships with the MCO's intake professionals in making a referral. This includes getting to know the individuals who perform the telephone intakes. Let's walk through the telephone intake process to better understand the EAP professional's role.

Telephone Intake

Most telephone intake procedures begin with gathering basic demographic information needed for registering the client. EAP professionals can facilitate the process by organizing the gathered information in the following way.

- Client's name
- Client's Social Security number
- Name of the primary insured
- Primary insured's Social Security number
- Client's address
- Client's phone number
- Name of employer group

Remember, MCOs are most likely to accept EAP professionals' assessments if they come across as partnering with MCO staff rather than as making demands.

As the intake continues, clinical information should be presented in behavioral terms. The information required would be:

- A brief description of the presenting problem
- A description of who is involved
- A list of professionals who may already be involved in the process

- A description of interventions that have been tried in the past
- A description of the expected goal of treatment
- A list of current medications
- Names of professionals who prescribed medication
- Known substance use and/or abuse

The only piece of the intake process that is left is getting a referral for continued care. EAP professionals who call in the intake information should let the MCO's intake coordinator know what requests they may have regarding the referral (i.e., gender, locale, or even specific provider by name). Because the MCOs, and not the EAPs, are usually financially at risk for the continued care, EAP professionals will find they are expected to accept the referral provided even if it is not their preferred choice. However, most often MCOs will try to accede to the request of the EAP professional.

Client Responsibility

EAP professionals should take responsibility for calling clients and informing them of the name and telephone number of the referred professional. Part of a successful interface protocol relies on EAP professionals not only to provide clients with the referral information, but also to perform a follow-up telephone call with clients two weeks later to make sure they are satisfied with the referral.

In the event that clients are not satisfied with their referrals, the protocol asks EAP professionals to change gears and refrain from acting for the client, and, instead, encourage them to contact the MCO themselves and get a new referral. At this point, EAP professionals are working in conjunction with the MCO agenda on getting clients to take responsibility for their own care.

Documentation

Once EAP professionals and MCO staff have mutually agreed upon the information for the interface protocol, EAP professionals should write out a document that explains the process and procedures. The explanation should include an outline of the aforementioned information, a list of contact people, and time guidelines for the procedure. In addition, EAP professionals should gather and take down names and telephone numbers of individuals to contact in case of a clinical emergency.

Both the MCOs and employer groups should be provided with a copy of this documentation because MCOs and EAP professionals share the same goal—to make good referrals so that clients get the appropriate clinical care at the right time—and part of the process is making sure that all parties are working from the same page.

CASE EXAMPLES

Sarah Is Not Doing Well

Sarah was referred to an EAP provider when she called the EAP referral line for her husband's company. Her husband's company had purchased a one- to three-session EAP program. In this program, the assessment sessions are prepaid by the employer so that there is nothing standing in the client's way to getting an assessment. When Sarah spoke to the EAP coordinator, she explained that she really did not know what her needs were, but she thought she was either having anxiety attacks or a reaction to the medication on which her primary care physician (PCP) had placed her. She told the intake coordinator that she was too embarrassed to call her PCP and wanted a referral for an assessment. Sarah was referred to a contracted EAP provider.

The EAP provider made an appointment to see Sarah within 48 hours. The therapist asked Sarah to explain why she had come to this assessment. Sarah stated that she had been feeling very anxious and she could not control the jittery feeling she was experiencing. She stated that this feeling had been constant since her PCP started her on an antianxiety medication approximately two weeks prior to this assessment. She was having difficulty describing all of her symptoms and became tearful. The therapist invited Sarah's husband into the session. He began to explain that Sarah had not done well since she started the medication. He stated that she could not think straight or sit still and that her skin seemed very itchy. As the conversation continued, the therapist quickly understood that Sarah needed to been seen by a psychiatrist for evaluation.

The EAP professional gathered all of the appropriate demographic information that was needed. The therapist then contacted the MCO that managed Sarah's mental health benefits. The EAP professional gave the MCO intake coordinator all of the information needed to get Sarah registered in their system (name, address, phone, Social Security number, etc.). Once Sarah was registered, the MCO intake coordinator asked the EAP professional to make a clinical recommendation.

The EAP professional explained the symptoms that Sarah had been experiencing. In addition, the EAP professional

explained Sarah and her husband's theory that her symptoms were caused by the antianxiety medication. Once the
clinical information was gathered and the diagnosis provided,
the EAP professional made the recommendation for an emergency psychiatric evaluation to assess the appropriateness of
Sarah's medication. The MCO intake coordinator asked the
EAP professional if he had a recommendation of a psychiatrist. The EAP professional suggested that he himself should
try a number of different panel psychiatrists to find out
which one had an immediate appointment. The EAP professional verified the names of the panel psychiatrists and told
the MCO intake coordinator that as soon as an appointment
was procured, the EAP professional would call the intake
specialist back with the name so that the authorization could
be generated.

The EAP professional called around to the various panel
psychiatrists. At the eighth call, the therapist found an appointment for Sarah the same afternoon. The therapist called
the MCO intake specialist back and received an authorization number to cover the medication evaluation. The EAP
professional gave Sarah the authorization number, the name
of the doctor, the appointment time, and directions to the
psychiatrist's office.

The EAP professional followed up with Sarah within a
few days. Sarah told the EAP professional that the psychiatrist had changed her medication and that she was already
starting to feel better. The EAP professional asked if Sarah
was happy with the referral. Sarah stated that she was. Finally, the EAP professional asked if Sarah felt she was in need
of any other service, such as psychotherapy. Sarah stated that
she did not feel that any additional services were needed.

Review

The EAP professionals need to assess the client's needs. In
this particular case, the EAP professional went above and

beyond the call of duty because the client was in a potentially emergent situation. The EAP professional felt that it was unsafe to leave the client to find her own referral since she was unable to articulate her needs. An assessment was made based on the information provided by the client and other available information. Finally, the EAP professional communicated with the MCO in a manner that allowed Sarah to get the services she needed when she needed them.

I Really Hate My Boss

Patricia was sitting in the lunchroom at her office. She looked up and saw the EAP poster reminding her to call if something was on her mind. Patricia called the toll-free number and told the EAP intake specialist that she was very stressed because she hated her boss and he had been particularly annoying on this day. Patricia found herself sitting in an EAP counselor's office the very next day. Patricia stated that she was very embarrassed as she had never been to counseling before. The EAP counselor explained that on this day they were really not doing counseling, but instead were going to assess what the problem was and refer Patricia to the proper treatment provider, if that was necessary.

Patricia explained that she was upset because she had worked for the same man for 10 years. Recently he retired from his role as the company's vice president and she became a personal secretary to a new boss, whom she did not like. She felt he was rude, and looked down on her. She explained his behaviors in detail. As she described the situation, and as the counselor asked information- gathering questions, Patricia began to hypothesize why her boss did what he did. In addition, she even began to reframe his behaviors as his way of doing business. She stated that her new boss had a good reputation for turning businesses around for the better, but that he had to be strict in order to achieve this. Patricia started to see his strictness as valuable and something she could work with if he set clear goals and boundaries.

She left the first EAP session, stating that it would be her last because she would now be too busy supporting her new boss' business strategies. A follow-up phone call two weeks later found the same response. Patricia felt that she had a purpose, and she felt that her relationship with her boss had improved. The EAP case was closed.

This outcome is not uncommon in EAP cases. Often the client needs to have a neutral place in which to brainstorm. The EAP session can provide the opportunity to talk about the situation in a new way. The result may be that additional services are necessary, and if this is the case, they should be coordinated by the EAP counselor. However, if the client states that no additional services are necessary, a simple follow-up will allow the EAP counselor once again to survey the client to ensure that case closure is appropriate.

Review

Counselors with EAPs should not get in the way of the client's success. Sometimes clients just need to have the space to investigate the problem from a different angle. In these cases, therapists should ask questions about the presenting problem that allow the client to explore freely and not get locked into a specific definition. In this particular case, the EAP counselor simply let Patricia find a way to view the problem differently so that it was no longer interpreted as a problem. The goal of an EAP is for both employee and employer to win. By purchasing an EAP, Patricia's company provided her with a resource that she may not have been inclined to seek out on her own. This opportunity created a venue for Patricia to reframe the situation. In turn, this produced a happier, healthier, and more productive employee.

The EAP professionals who establish solid interface protocols find themselves in a win–win situation. As can be seen in these cases, the provider aligns with both the MCO and the client. Providing excellent clinical care leaves the client feeling satisfied. The goal of MCOs is to have their client's satisfied and to promote and provide excellent quality of care. A strong interface protocol can showcase the providers' strong suites, which in all likelihood will lead to a larger referral base from the MCOs.

4

Brief Philosophies

If you were to talk to a therapist who works from a brief therapy modality, it would become apparent that the therapist was very aligned with the MCOs' philosophies. Therapists who work from brief modalities find that they rarely have a treatment plan amended and they find few limitations impeding their work. Although all brief therapy modalities have value when working with managed care cases, the most successful are those that are systemic in nature. This chapter looks at the therapies of the Mental Research Institute (MRI) and solution-focused therapy and how they make a good marriage with managed care.

THE MRI APPROACH

MRI operates from a behavioral rather than a semantic model of therapy. The theory of MRI is based on the concept that the client/family gets stuck in an unsuccessful solution pattern that is assumed to maintain the presenting problem (Watzlawick, Weakland, & Fisch, 1974).

The goals of the initial session are to gain a clear definition of the presenting problem, obtain an understanding of the solutions previously attempted, identify who is involved in the problem, and define the smallest sign of change the family would accept as a sign that greater change could occur (Fisch, Weakland, & Segal, 1982).

The MRI therapist tracks the attempted solutions by asking questions to obtain the outlined information and then prescribes an intervention (either direct or paradoxical). The intervention is designed to disrupt the cycle of the attempted solutions the clients have tried and retried but that do not work.

The goal of the therapy is to help the client identify goals in behavioral terms and find new ways to move toward those goals. This approach helps the client/family to find relief from the problem in a time-sensitive manner. In order to achieve this goal, the MRI therapist puts the client/family in the expert role by taking a one-down position in order to maintain greater maneuverability (Fisch, Weakland, & Segal, 1982).

The original MRI research showed that most clients found relief from their symptoms in an average of seven sessions (Watzlawick, Weakland, & Fisch, 1974). In addition, the literature (Weakland, Fisch, Watzlawick, & Bodin, 1974; Garfield and Bergin , 1978; Koss, 1979; de Shazer, 1985) shows that the average number of sessions in which the client/family stays engaged in treatment is seven. This same literature shows that the client reports resolution to the presenting problem in this small number of therapy sessions.

For these reasons, it would seem likely that the therapist would want to work in the most efficacious way with the estimated number of sessions in which the client/family is expected to stay engaged.

As managed care companies began to mature, it became apparent that the charge of managing benefits could not be an easy task (Poynter, 1994). Simply denying care to meet the demanding limits of new benefit packages did not make good sense clinically, ethically, or morally. Therefore, this forced the MCOs to look at clinically sound treatment modalities that provided quality care, reduced problem symptoms, and was time sensitive. The MRI approach, in addition to other systemic modalities, works well within the managed care setting.

The following clinical cases exemplify the use of MRI therapy in the managed care setting.

CASE EXAMPLES

He Only Feels Sorry for Me

Sandy was a 50-year-old woman. She accessed her benefits when she moved into town. She had a history of psychiatric treatment and hospitalizations. When she came to therapy, she presented with her husband of one year. She came to treatment because she was "depressed," had suffered a lot of abuse in her previous marriage, and felt that her current husband had only married her because he felt sorry for her. The goals of therapy were to help the client stay stabilized on medications since she reported having had success with the medications in the past. The next goal was to have conjoint sessions with the husband so that they could work on communication about the past abuse and learn how to be different in this marriage in order that Sandy could learn not to judge her current husband based on her experiences with her first husband. Sandy stated that she "suffered from poor self-esteem due to the past abuse." The abuse lasted for the greater portion of Sandy's life and the effects would not go away quickly. Therefore, the therapist believed that trying to "cure" Sandy's self-esteem problem would be too big a goal to tackle (Shilts & Gordon, 1993). Instead, the therapist helped the client to identify the smallest sign of change that would let her know that her self-esteem was improving and would continue to improve.

The therapist described in the treatment plan that first the couple and therapist clearly defined the problem, and second, they defined who was involved in the problem. The couple both agreed that the people who were involved were themselves. They did not have any children in the home, all relatives lived in other states, and being new to the geographic area, they did not have friends there. Neither had any contact with the former spouses nor did want to have any. They agreed that the solution that they had attempted took the form of Sandy's husband trying to convince her that he loved her by saying so over and over again. Their stuck solution pattern looked something like this:

Husband says, "I love you."

Sandy gets more depressed   Sandy believes he is lying
and despondent.   to make her feel better.

Husband swears that he
loves Sandy.

Sandy continued in treatment with her husband. The treatment goals were to have the husband find many different ways to say "I love you" and not to overreact when Sandy became depressed and despondent. In addition, Sandy was to find different ways to "test" her husband other than becoming despondent.

Because the couple would occasionally get stuck in their old pattern, sessions were spread out in order to give them practice time. The most important thing the couple learned was that their stuck solution pattern did not need to destroy them or their relationship. The hardest thing for them to remember was that many of their problems were based on reactions from past relationships. However, they intellectually understood that they could not change the past relationships and that it would take time to correct their learned habits. Upon review of the treatment summary, the therapist stated that the goals had been achieved.

With this in mind, the couple would often check out of therapy when things were going well and then would come back if they got stuck again. They did this approximately three times over a two-year time span. Each time the couple came back they had made progress and did not get stuck in the same place. The last time they reinitiated counseling, they were able to identify that their behaviors were what lead to their getting stuck.

At each step of the way, the therapist communicated to the MCO. First, the therapist communicated a comprehensive treatment plan that included the husband; the therapist had immediately recognized that the solution resided between both spouses. This allowed the couple to feel some immediate relief from their presenting problem. Had the therapist simply bought into the concept that Sandy had emotional problems, the problem might have been perpetuated. Second, the therapist updated the MCO case manager as to the progress that the couple was making. The MCO case manager came to have confidence in the therapist as behavioral improvement could be seen and measured. This ability to quantify progress is an important key to obtaining preferred standing with MCOs.

The better the therapy is outlined and goals are measured, the greater confidence case managers will have in the care that the therapist provides. This is significant as many MCOs move toward programs in which they do not manage their core providers. MCOs that are interested in designing such programs will review practice patterns to see if the therapist can fit the program. Well-documented treatment plans and treatment summaries will help to show the therapist's practice pattern.

Is My Granddaughter in Danger?

When Elizabeth called to set her first appointment, she stated that she was in crisis and feeling extremely anxious. During the first session, she reported to the therapist that for many years during her childhood, she had been sexually abused by her grandfather. Elizabeth became very tearful as she told her story. She then asked if she could bring her husband into the session for support.

When asked why this was more of a problem now than in the past, she stated that her daughter recently had a child. When her daughter's marriage did not thrive, Elizabeth's daughter and granddaughter moved into Elizabeth's home. Elizabeth stated that she had recently read an article in the newspaper that said that adults who were abused are more likely to abuse children than adults who were not abused. This concerned Elizabeth because she did not want to inflict the type of pain she had endured on another child.

During the first session, Elizabeth was full of questions.

She wanted to know if she should have her daughter and granddaughter move out. Should she not baby-sit for her granddaughter? Did she need to have a chaperone around when she saw her granddaughter? How could she learn to trust herself? After hearing all of Elizabeth's questions, the therapist began to ask Elizabeth some questions. The therapist inquired about who else was concerned about her hurting her granddaughter. What had she done to assure them that she would not hurt her granddaughter? What would need to happen to convince her that she did not have a problem?

These questions confused Elizabeth because she had expected to hear that she had a long-standing problem and would always need to keep the people she loved at bay. The therapist began to reframe Elizabeth's fears as her way of caring for her granddaughter. The therapist questioned Elizabeth about whether or not she had abused her daughter. Before Elizabeth could respond, her husband vigorously stated that she had never done such a thing. Elizabeth also stated that she had never harmed her daughter. The therapist then asked if Elizabeth's daughter had ever been abused by anyone else. Both Elizabeth and her husband stated that their daughter had never been abused. They were curious as to why the therapist had asked.

The therapist then asked them how they were able to keep their daughter protected in a very dangerous world. They stated that they always checked the references of people with whom she was left and at an early age taught her about safety. The therapist asked why Elizabeth felt that she would harm her granddaughter when she had not harmed her daughter. Elizabeth then referenced the article she had read in the newspaper. The therapist helped to reframe the situation (Piercy & Sprenkle, 1986) by pointing out that the article stated that most individuals who abuse children have been found to have been abused as children. Although the article alluded to the fact that if a person had been abused, there was a greater likelihood that that person would abuse another, the therapist pointed out that there was a gap in the article's theory. What was missing from the article was that there are many individuals who have experienced and yet have not gone on to become abusers. The logic of the article was one-sided. And, Elizabeth was an example of the side not addressed.

The therapist reported to the MCO case manager that the client had begun to find new meaning in her anxiety and fear. She understood that she loved her granddaughter and only wanted her to be safe and happy. In just one session, Elizabeth had started to feel better. She and her husband attended only two more sessions. Over the course of those two sessions, Elizabeth reported that she felt less anxious and fearful. She left therapy knowing that she knew how to keep children safe and that she could enjoy her family.

MRI therapy effects change in various ways, most prominently in behavior and perception. The MRI approach facilitates the ability to do something different, to become "unstuck," breaking the pattern of futile solution attempts. Another way to effect change is to help the individuals find new meanings in their behaviors. This is known as reframing. When clients learn to reframe their situations, they look at problems differently and often learn that what they had identified as the problem is not really a problem at all.

Because of its therapeutic processes, MRI therapy helps to create change in a family system in a short time. This form of therapy is a natural marriage with managed mental health care in that it allows individuals to develop appropriate strategies for solving their problems. In addition, it allows for symptom relief within a brief period, which also means that individuals get the most coverage from their insurance benefits.

problems, they just may not remember that they know (de Shazer et al., 1986). With this in mind, therapists query about when the problem is not a problem and then build on the client's experiences of success. This step allows the client to focus on finding solutions as opposed to focusing only on the problem itself.

An example of such refocusing might be when the parents of a young child come to therapy stating that their son is always acting out and cannot be controlled. In solution-focused therapy, the focus of the therapy will be the family, not the individual child. The therapist will ask the family to describe the times when the young child is not acting out. The following excerpt* shows this approach in action.

Therapist: What portion of the day is Tommy in control?

Mother: Well, he's good when he sleeps. Actually he is an angel when he sleeps.

Therapist: Let me understand this. He sleeps how many hours out of each day?

Mother: Oh, he's a good sleeper; he sleeps nine hours a night.

Therapist: Okay, now we need to look at the other 16 hours of the day. During these 16 hours, does Tommy act out for the entire time or are there times that you can control him?

Tommy: My teacher says that I am good in school.

Mother: This is true; he always gets good scores in behavior. And the teacher has never complained about his being uncontrollable.

------

*This dialogue is from a videotaped session of the author while she was working in a training environment and is shared with client's consent.

THE SOLUTION-FOCUSED APPROACH

Solution-focused treatment was developed by the Brief Family Therapy Center (BFTC) in Milwaukee (de Shazer, Berg, Lipchick, Nunnaly, Molnar, Gingerich, & Weiner-Davis, 1986). Initially based on the theory of MRI, the BFTC took the therapy one step further. The therapists realized that they could obtain a great deal of clinical information by asking the client/family about when the problem was not a problem. The therapists at BFTC began their therapy by first gaining an understanding of the presenting problem and then immediately initializing questioning with the family about when things were going well (de Shazer, 1985; de Shazer et al., 1986). This seemed to cause a shift in the client's thinking and the BFTC therapists found that the client/families quickly moved on to naming solutions to the problems.

This led to the idea that client/families had less of a problem to deal with than they had originally thought. De Shazer et al. (1986) explained the idea this way:

> The key to brief therapy is utilizing what clients bring with them to help them meet their needs in such a way that they can make satisfactory lives for themselves. (p. 208)

Utilizing this approach, solution-focused therapists help the clients/families to view the situations differently so that obstacles to finding solutions to their problems are addressed early on.

In order to accomplish this, therapists need to ask clients how they might get more positive results and the clients are guided to construct solutions. It is important for therapists to remember that clients already own the skills to solve their

Therapist: Okay, let me see if I understand this. Tommy is in school for seven hours every day and is in control. Now we need to focus on only nine hours every weekday and more on the weekends. During these times, is Tommy out of control all the time?

Mother: No, Tommy behaves some of the time, but when I want him to, he just doesn't listen. It's probably just a few hours each day.

Therapist: Are there other times you are able to have Tommy behave, or, as you say to control him. Umm, how do you do that, keep him in control, I mean?

Mother: I set rules and expect him to follow them, and I give him privileges based on his ability to follow rules.

The mother was able to shift from stating that Tommy was always out of control to finding specific times when Tommy was out of control. In addition, she was able to document for herself and the therapist that there were times that she could control Tommy and had had success in this area. In more traditional forms of therapy, the therapist might pathologize the child, placing him in individual therapy and checking in with the parents after each session to explain the child's problem and progress.

As managed care organizations learned more about brief therapy, they realized that solution-oriented approaches were effective with the majority of the population that they served. Like MRI, solution-focused therapy allows clients to find symptom relief in a time-sensitive fashion that allows the MCOs to utilize the client's benefits wisely. However, when the child is identified as the problem, the form of treatment which allows the child to be pathologized can be more costly, more time-consuming, and most probably a less effective form of therapy.

CASE EXAMPLES

Jimmy Turns the Lights Out

Jimmy's parents contacted the MCO in order to activate mental health benefits and receive a referral for counseling. Jimmy was a 15-year-old boy who lived with his biological parents. He had an older brother, who was away at college. In the initial phone call, the parents stated that Jimmy had been involved with the courts due to a "minor situation."

At the first session, Jimmy stated that he did not have a problem. When the parents were asked what they viewed the problem to be, they stated that they, too, were convinced that the "incident" Jimmy was accused of was really a misinterpretation. The therapist asked for a clearer description of the incident. The parents were hesitant about speaking in front of Jimmy, but the therapist pointed out that Jimmy was the one involved and that surely he already knew what happened.

The therapist then asked Jimmy to explain. Jimmy stated that he was jogging and saw a woman struggling with her groceries. He stopped to help her, and when they went into the elevator, she got nervous about allowing a stranger to help. When the elevator stopped, she ran out without her groceries. This scared Jimmy, who ran down the stairs and took a bike so that he could get away fast. He was picked up by the police for stealing a bike. The parents believed Jimmy's story and went through a local court mediation and arbitration program; the outcome was for the family to go to therapy.

At this time, the therapist had a number of options. One would be to see Jimmy on his own in order to discuss ways to satisfy the court program. The therapist could have believed that Jimmy's making light of the situation meant that he was in denial. In addition, the therapist could have reified that Jimmy had a problem in the eyes of the parents.

Another option would be for the therapist to work from the treatment modality of seeing the family together and finding ways to improve the strained relationship. The therapist chose to work this way and in a solution-focused manner. The treatment plan consisted of clearly defined goals for improving parent–child communication, demonstrated by a better understanding of the statements made; helping the parents to work together to make decisions that affected their son, as evidenced by holding private discussions before decisions are made; and the son's being given age-appropriate responsibilities based on those given to others in his peer group and his ability to handle them emotionally.

At first, the parents and son were opposed to conjoint therapy. The parents felt that if a problem existed, it resided in Jimmy. The therapist explained to the parents that therapy was not about finding fault. In a joking fashion, it was explained that the insurance company would not pay for assigning blame. Instead, the goal of meeting together was to find mutually accepted solutions so that the family could move forward and have solutions on hand if other problems should arise. They all agreed to this plan of action. The treatment plan was then submitted to the MCO. A medication evaluation was not necessary. The MCO case manager approved of the treatment plan, and further sessions were authorized. The therapist estimated the length of treatment to be six to eight sessions.

During the first session, it became apparent to the therapist that this family did not have much experience in talking to one another. The parents were somewhat guarded and often uncomfortable, and at other times they would be brutally honest about Jimmy's shortcomings. Jimmy did not verbalize his anger, but found other ways to let people know. When he left the session, he vandalized the emergency electrical switch, which turned the electricity off in the entire building. This was particularly significant since this was the switch the fire department would use if there were a fire in the building. This gesture took on greater meaning because Jimmy's father was chief of a local fire department.

It was unknown at the time of the second session that Jimmy was the cause of the blackout. The father and Jimmy showed up at the second session alone. In this session, the father reported that he and his wife were working better as a team. He stated that they spent much time discussing the last session. The therapist spent some time alone with Jimmy to get his perception of the situation. He stated that his parents did not listen to him or to each other and that he had become used to being left alone. He reported that he only got attention when he was in trouble.

Jimmy and his father were asked to book their next appointment when the mother could be there with them. As the father stood in the front office to make his appointment, the electricity went out again, and he joked with the front office staff that the office had " bad karma."

A worker from an adjoining office saw Jimmy break the switch and came into the therapy office to get his name. The therapist questioned a few other people in order to make sure it had been Jimmy. The therapist stated that he could not give out Jimmy's identity because he had to assure confidentiality, but that he would address the situation.

The therapist called the father and mother and explained what had happened. They both stated that the therapist must have been mistaken. The therapist used this situation to help the parents with their treatment plan. The therapist asked the parents to come in for a session without Jimmy. They did, and during the session, the therapist helped them to discuss what had happened, derive a meaning from the event, and decide on a plan of action for discussing the situation with Jimmy and making him pay restitution.

The parents went home and sat Jimmy down for a talk. They reported that they told him he had been caught breaking the electrical switch and that there was no excuse for his behavior. In addition, they explained the potential damage that could have been incurred, and what they expected from him now. The father stated that they would pay the bill for repairs, but that Jimmy had to pay them back by helping to paint the house and helping with repairs around the house for the next four weekends. The parents then used the time together to become reacquainted with their son, to gain an understanding of what he could and could not handle emotionally, and to find positive things about which to compliment him.

The therapist filed a termination summary that stated the total number of sessions (four), the original presenting problem (incident involving the local police department), the prognosis (good, in that the parents had learned to better communicate with each other and their son), the reports given to the court (informed the court that treatment was completed), and future plans if further therapy was needed (the therapist explained to the parents that they should call the MCO if any additional care was necessary down the line).

Follow-up

Jimmy's relationship with his parents improved drastically at a critical stage in his life. He learned how to communicate with his parents and to use them as a resource instead of viewing them as adversaries. Two years after the initial incident, the mother called the MCO to get a referral for Jimmy to see a drug counselor. Jimmy freely admitted to his parents that he was "hanging around some kids who smoked pot and he did some too." He went to his parents and asked for help to stop because he did not want to "get into the drug scene." His parents responded appropriately, by complimenting him on his decision and his coming to them for help. They decided to call the MCO for a referral. At the last report from Jimmy's father, Jimmy was doing well in treatment, and his parents were also involved.

What did the therapist do that convinced the MCO case manager that he had an appropriate treatment plan? First, he was aware of the fact that the problem was systemic and documented it accordingly. He did not buy into the idea that the problem resided in Jimmy. He communicated to the MCO the parents' initial resistance and a comprehensive treatment plan that addressed it. Second, the therapist helped the parents find a clear definition of the problem so that they would be able to identify signs of change. Third, the therapist utilized the situation at hand to show the parents pragmatic tools to use so as not to fall back into the trap of placing the fault with Jimmy. Fourth, the therapist aided the parents in finding solutions that could be applied to other situations with Jimmy and his older brother as well. Finally, the therapist explained that the family might need some help in the future, and that if they ever did, they should call the MCO for a referral.

Psychotic Episodes Again and Again

Mandy was brought into a local emergency room when her blood sugar level rose to extreme proportions after she did not take her medication for her chronic diabetes. While in the emergency room, Mandy became combative, and before long it was realized that she was delusional and had a history of psychosis. Mandy was admitted to a psychiatric unit in a medical hospital so that she could be stabilized on insulin and antipsychotic medication.

After being stabilized and released from the hospital, she was assigned to a therapist* who worked from a solution-focused modality. The therapist submitted an initial treatment plan that discussed the need to engage the husband in treatment and that the client was not a suitable candidate for exploring psychological issues. Instead, the goal of therapy was to be education about the diagnosis, how to identify signs that the client was slipping, and simple solutions to keep things as normal as possible.

These types of cases pose great difficulty to the MCO because they are so costly and time consuming. There are a number of reasons for this. First, the process of inpatient stabilization gets longer with each relapse that the client experiences (Goldberg & Harrow, 1994). The client has a limited number of inpatient days, and if the client uses all the budgeted inpatient days, he/she will more than likely be re-hospitalized in a community facility. This often moves the coordination of care out of the control of the MCO, and discharge planning becomes nearly impossible to coordinate. Second, the client has a limited number of outpatient visits and the majority of them will be used for the psychiatrist and/or home health care, which leaves an even more limited number of sessions for therapy.

During the first session, the therapist established that the client and her family did not understand her diagnosis and how it affected the family. Nor did they understand the signs that she was decompensating. The therapist determined that they were eager to be a part of her care but they did not know

---

*Jimmy Rudes, Ph.D., LMFT, a private practitioner in Hollywood, Florida. Dr. Rudes is currently on the panel of a number of MCOs and is an adjunct professor at Barry University in Miami.

how. In addition, the family did not know how to access the resources that were available to them.

Initially, the therapist spent most of his time trying to build rapport with Mandy so that she would not need to feel paranoid around him. The therapist understood early in the process that he was going to be a therapeutic coach. He had Mandy and her husband sign information releases so that he could speak with the MCO and the psychiatrist.

Once in communication with the MCO case manager, the therapist explained that Mandy's benefits would best be used for medication management. The therapist explained that Mandy was still not understanding the importance of staying on her medication. Furthermore, the therapist explained that the psychiatrist was not confident that Mandy would keep her medication management appointment. This information allowed the MCO case manager to put solutions in place that would work in Mandy's favor. With the help of the psychiatrist, the MCO case manager arranged for a home health care agency to go to Mandy's home twice monthly to give her the medication in injection form. Finally, the case manager spoke with Mandy's husband about opening a case in his name, since family therapy was the primary modality, and explained the need to save Mandy's sessions for medication management. Mandy's husband agreed.

With all of the above in place, the therapist was free to stay focused on therapy and find ways for Mandy and her husband to find solutions. The therapist began by finding out within what areas Mandy could be organized. Mandy and her husband explained that they had three small children in the home. Except during her worst psychosis, Mandy was able to take care of the children and organize herself around their needs. She stated that this was a great love of hers and that the children gave her strength.

The therapist began to build the metaphor that the children "were a real island of health." The therapist started a line of questioning that helped Mandy and her husband understand that although the children were small, they could still help to keep Mandy healthy. In addition, Mandy stated she would want to be healthy for her children. Until this time, Mandy did not see value in medication. When she began to understand that the medication would keep her "calmer," Mandy agreed to have someone from the home health care agency come to her house to give her the injections.

The family sessions were spread out over the months. Mandy and her husband were seen every two to three weeks by the therapist. During this time, Mandy's husband learned how to identify the early signs of relapse. A plan was in place for the husband to report to Mandy when he saw these signs and for Mandy to contact the therapist. The therapist worked with Mandy to understand that this was part of her "healthy life plan." Mandy now viewed the therapist, the psychiatrist, the MCO, the home health care agency, and her family as all part of the same team, and one of which she did not need to be frightened.

The therapist built on solutions that were already familiar to Mandy and her family. This allowed Mandy and her family to utilize the resources that they already had and to add to them. The solution-focused approach provided the client and her family with a therapeutic environment that granted her greater chances of remaining stable.

Many therapists may be skeptical about using a solution-focused approach when a client has such a severe diagnosis. However, the therapist must keep in mind the ultimate goal—to keep the client stable on medication, to educate the client and the client's family about the diagnosis, and to find ways to prevent relapse while still maintaining a "normal" life. After all, when the client decompensates, it causes more anguish for the client and the family.

Follow-up

Mandy and her family still remain in therapy. The family is doing well and have been successful in identifying potential relapse. Mandy had one close call this past year, but her husband was able to identify the early warning signs and Mandy contacted the therapist. The therapist immediately called the team together as he promised he would. This allowed Mandy to get her medications recalibrated and she avoided hospitalization. For the first time in seven years, Mandy was not hospitalized.

SUMMARY

The brief systemic therapies of MRI and solution-focused allow for symptom reduction in a short period of time. These therapies are based in "wellness" and utilize the client's resources to introduce new behaviors, or new ways to think about the presenting problem. Family therapists working from these modalities are primed to enter into or to continue a productive relationship with MCOs. MCOs need to balance the scales between cost-effective care and sound clinical care. For this reason, therapists who are not familiar with these modalities should obtain education and certification. Therapists who are well versed in these modalities should highlight this on the application for panelship of MCOs. Therapists who work from these modalities and are already on MCO panels need only wait until their work proves their value to the organization.

5

The Strategic, Structural, and Milan Approaches

This chapter continues the discussion of brief therapies and how they fit into the managed care philosophy. Various family therapies are touched on and how they can be applied to cases managed by MCOs is discussed. This chapter also looks at case examples to show "do's" and don'ts" in managed care.

THE STRATEGIC APPROACH

One problem that may arise that MCOs may not even be conscious of at this time is making the identified patient (IP) a minor child. Very often the parent will call to initiate care and will state that the minor child has a problem. More often than not, the problem is a parent–child problem and the care can be just as easily conducted under the umbrella of the parent's case. Of course, if the child has a major psychiatric problem that requires the use of psychotropic medications, then a medical records chart must be opened for the minor child. However, unnecessary diagnoses for children may imply preexisting conditions that will cause difficulty for them in later years when they attempt to acquire health and life insurance.

In either instance, the primary goal of treatment should be for the therapist to provide family therapy. It is unlikely that the therapist can effect change in the child without the intimate involvement of the adults living with the child (Haley, 1976; Madanes, 1981); after all, the child does not live in a vacuum. Too often, the adults will opt to "drop off" the child at the therapist's office and to pick up the child an hour later. In these cases, the parents most often have the unspoken goal of retrieving a "cured" child. Family therapists do not buy into this model and therefore foster greater behavioral and semantic change more rapidly than do therapists with individual therapy. The goal of strategic therapy is to realign the family structure, utilizing the resources that the family already owns. The therapist utilizes maneuverability and paradox (Haley, 1976) to help the family to find a healthier way of being.

The review of cases often shows various types of family therapy modalities that fit well with the philosophies of MCOs. Strategic therapy, the major proponents of which are Jay Haley (1976) and Cloe Madanes (1980), allows great maneuverability of the therapist, especially in cases that involve children and adolescents. Both Haley and Madanes find that problems are perpetuated by a faulty hierarchy within the family. The goal of strategic family therapy is to change the family's interactions, which in turn change the family's structure to produce healthier relationships. In addition, they maintain that the presenting problem is often a metaphor for the actual problem (Haley, 1976; Madanes, 1981). For example, a family may report that the young child has been experiencing strong school phobias. A more detailed evaluation of the problem may reveal that the mother has recently returned to work and that the young child goes to day care when school is over. Not liking the after-school program, the child began to have tantrums as he started off for school each day, and the first few times that this occurred, the mother stayed home with him. This shift in power is what strategic family therapists look for.

The strategic family therapist will often align himself/herself with the parental generation when dealing with child-focused problems (Haley, 1980). The goal of strategic therapy is to bring parents together to work on their child's problems. Aside from realigning problematic hierarchies, this therapy also can serve to strengthen the parental relationship. Strategic family therapy is structured to alter malfunctioning triangles (Haley, 1976, 1980) and incongruent hierarchies (Madanes, 1980, 1981) using such diverse interventions as reframing, paradox, "pretending," ordeals, and unbalancing through creating alternative coalitions. In the example just provided, the therapist also may have uncovered the fact that the father was not very happy about his wife's returning to work. Therefore, the young child was acting out the father's dissatisfaction. An intervention may focus on having the father and son plan to make the mother's lunch each day. This would help the father and son to find a way to the support each other as they learn to support the mother's choices as well.

To summarize the main points of this approach, strategic family therapy:

- *Is indirect and confrontive.* In this example, the therapist would confront the parents, letting them see that they need to support each other's decisions in order to help their son be comfortable with their decisions.

- *Emphasizes the importance of maladaptive behavioral sequences in dysfunction.* The therapist would explain that the son's behavior was a metaphor for the problems of adapting to change within a family.

- *Emphasizes positive feedback cycles.* The therapist would explain to the mother that each time she stayed home with her young child, she rewarded his behavior.

- *Presupposes that the therapist often works with only one or two members of a family system.* The therapist would most likely work with the mother and father to strengthen their parental and couple relationship. The idea is that when the mother and father agree on how to handle the situation, the young child no longer will have a need to act out.

- *Emphasizes out-of-session directives.* The therapist would ask the couple to act out an intervention during the time between sessions. In this case, the therapist may ask the father to act out the lunch intervention. When the couple returns to treatment, the therapist will look at the difference that the intervention has produced.

As mentioned earlier, this form of therapy can be a good match to the philosophies of the MCOs. Strategic family therapy can have long-lasting effects in a brief time. The following case scenarios exemplify how strategic family therapy can be applied in the MCO setting.

CASE EXAMPLES

But Her Mother Died

Tracy called to initiate mental health care for her 9-year-old niece, Lisa, whom she recently adopted. Lisa's mother had died from cancer four months earlier, and Lisa moved to her aunt and uncle's home. They already had two children, and another was on the way. Lisa, who had been an only child living with her single mother, was now thrown into a new family with siblings while still adjusting to her mother's death. Two months after moving in, she and her new family moved from the northeastern United States to southern Florida.

Tracy was concerned that Lisa was not adjusting well and wanted to bring her to therapy so that she would have someone to talk to. Tracy was asked to bring all the household members to the first therapy session. She agreed. Four days later, Tracy, her husband Michael, and the three children came to meet the therapist. During the first session, Tracy restated the recent history to the therapist and reiterated that she felt that Lisa needed someone to talk to. The therapist quickly reframed the concept that Lisa needed to speak to the therapist alone. When the therapist asked Tracy what her rule in the household was about talking to strangers, she said that she tells the children that they are not allowed to speak to strangers. The therapist then explained that as she was a stranger to the children, they would probably be more comfortable if Tracy and her husband were present.

Tracy still was concerned that Lisa had "pent-up feelings over her mother's death." The therapist questioned the family with regard to who was the confidante in the family. Tracy reported that she was the one to whom everyone came when they had a problem. The therapist followed that line of questioning and found out that Lisa would also go to Tracy when she needed to discuss something. Tracy would take all major decisions to a family meeting. During the family meetings, Lisa would often start crying and have a tantrum when she did not get her way. She inevitably would mention how her mother had allowed her to do as she pleased.

The therapist spoke with Tracy and Michael about how difficult it is to raise someone else's child. They agreed that they had had a difficult time setting limits, and were concerned that they would upset Lisa more if they set limits that were too strict. After speaking to Lisa about her mother for a few minutes, the therapist determined that she was going through the normal adjustment period and needed to settle in to new routines.

The therapist developed a treatment plan that helped to define the parental hierarchy (Haley, 1980), and still maintain the confidence in Tracy that Lisa had developed. In addition, there was the goal to decrease the number of temper tantrums that Lisa had when she did not get her way. The therapist began by having a meeting with Tracy and Michael to educate them about the grief process that Lisa might go through. It was explained that they needed to be sensitive to Lisa's situation, but that they did not need to give in to her just because of her tragedy. Tracy's special understanding of Lisa, due to her own experience of loss–that of her sister— was then discussed.

Tracy was given a homework task (Haley, 1976). She was to find a bit of time each day in which to talk to Lisa about her mother. If Lisa should come up with a request, Tracy was to explain that she needed to discuss the issue with Michael. Tracy would give Lisa a timeframe within which she would give her a reply. After talking with Michael and coming to a solution, the two would present the answer to Lisa conjointly and privately. No matter what her response, they were to maintain their position.

During the next session, Tracy and Michael reported that they had implemented the new communication pattern. They reported that it helped to decrease the number of tantrums, once Lisa learned that she could not split them. Tracy also reported that having an opportunity to remember her sister with Lisa helped her to understand that she need not be nervous about Lisa's grief process.

They practiced this technique over the next few weeks. The couple reported that things had improved tremendously. Tracy and Michael even used this new method with their own daughter. They found that this helped to make Michael less peripheral, and that the girls even started to go to him first at times.

The family attended a total of six sessions and the case was closed. Why does this case fit the managed care environment so well? First, the therapist worked with the strengths of the family. The therapist did not try to pathologize the IP and instead looked for the interrelational patterns that caused problems for the family. Second, the therapist designed the least intrusive treatment plan. Simply stated, this means that the therapist clearly defined the presenting problems and stayed focused on finding solutions to these problems. Third, the therapist utilized the family's resources and willingness to try interventions at home. Finally, the therapist did not move into a hand-holding mode for Lisa and instead allowed the family to do this for her.

Follow-up

The family reinitiated treatment one year later for a total of four sessions. The main focus of this treatment was Tracy's concern that she was not understanding the girls as they moved into adolescence. A brief treatment goal of developmental education and reinstatement of communication skills was set by a new therapist. When working with MCOs, it is important to find out information about past therapies. Although you may not want the old work to creep into the new, you may also find resources that the client may have forgotten about. In this case, the current therapist obtained a release of information from the client to speak to the previous therapist. This gave the new therapist great resources to work with, which in turn allowed the family to be in therapy for even a shorter time.

The Kids Are Acting Up Again

Katherine called the MCO for a referral to see a therapist because she could no longer stop her children from acting out. Katherine and her three children attended the first session. In the first session, she stated that the children were continuously fighting with one another and often became physical in their fights. During the first session, each one of the children tried to get the attention of the therapist by yelling, standing on the chair, or pushing another child out of the way. Since the first session was so chaotic, the therapist asked Katherine to come to the next session with only her husband (the children's stepfather). The therapist contacted the MCO and asked for an extension on the assessment authorization. The therapist explained that the first session was so chaotic that he was unable to gather all the information needed to complete the diagnostic assessment and treatment plan.

During the second session, Katherine explained that her first husband had physically abused her and the children. She stated that she had to run away from the family home in order to survive. She left in the middle of the night with the children and stayed in a shelter until she could get a restraining order to keep her husband away from the house so that she could move back in. She went on to explain that even after she was officially divorced, her ex-husband had difficulty letting go and had actually set her house on fire. She stated that the children were terrified of their father, but that she did not like to talk about it with them as she felt she would upset them.

The therapist turned to the stepfather and asked him what his thoughts were on this. He stated that he and Katherine always argued about it because he feels that the children do need to talk about their father. He thought that they were acting out because their mother always found something else to do rather than to sit down and talk with them. He further hypothesized that Katherine did not want to talk about the past, not only because it was painful, but because she did not want to burden him.

The therapist asked the couple how the children did in school. Both parents reported that the children did well and only one of them had some behavioral problems. The middle child (David) had difficulty staying seated and focusing on the teacher.

The therapist devised a treatment plan that allowed for the family to discuss what they had all experienced and what their fears were. The therapist, Katherine, and the stepfather designed family meetings that they could hold nightly for approximately 30 minutes. The therapist stated the goals of therapy would be to assess the outcomes of the family meetings, improve the behaviors of the children by improving the communication that provided them with feedback as to what their behavior meant, and to improve the parental relationship by having the parents share the responsibilities of the children.

The entire family came to the third session. The therapist asked about the family meetings. The children stated that they liked the meetings and were happy that they all had an opportunity to sit down and talk. The stepfather said that he was surprised that at some point during every meeting, Katherine would leave to go to the bathroom. Embarrassed, Katherine asked if the children would leave the therapy room. When they left, Katherine became very agitated and explained that she was abusing laxatives to control her weight. A secondary gain was that she could easily (or most often needed to) run to the bathroom to get away from the discussions, which she found very upsetting. She did say that she was very pleased that the children's behavior had improved during the week and that was the reason she gave for wanting to stop using the laxatives. She stated that she knew she did not have to hide from this anymore.

The therapist asked Katherine to see her primary care physician (PCP) to have a physical and design a way to safely stop using the laxatives. The therapist had Katherine sign a release of information so that the therapist could speak to the PCP. In addition, the therapist discussed with Katherine how she could be a part of the family meetings. The therapist put an intervention in place—that the stepfather would call the meetings spontaneously, and preferably at a different time each day. This would help prevent Katherine from getting worked up about the meetings and not allow her the lead time to take the laxatives.

The therapist contacted the MCO to inform the case manager that the treatment plan had been altered, and explained the changes in the plan. In addition, the therapist contacted the PCP in order to coordinate care. The PCP reported that Katherine was in good health, but that she did need to stop the use of laxatives before it became dangerous. The PCP explained to the therapist the type of physical complaints that Katherine would probably experience so that the therapist would be prepared.

Katherine and her family returned for a total of 10 sessions. The family sessions helped the children and Katherine to put the past behind them. Katherine and the stepfather reported that the children's behavior improved. Katherine said that had she stopped using laxatives. The stepfather reported that he felt that he was now a part of the family and felt needed. Katherine did report that David still was experiencing problems in school. Given his symptoms and the fact that the previous interventions did not change his school problems, the therapist suggested a consultation with the psychiatrist. The parents agreed.

The therapist contacted the MCO one more time and consulted with the case manager. They agreed that a psychiatric evaluation was appropriate to have an assessment to rule out attention-deficit/ hyperactivity disorder (ADHD). The case manager gave the therapist the name of a child psychiatrist, the psychiatrist's office phone number, and an authorization number. The therapist passed this information on to Katherine and had her sign a release of information so that the therapist could contact the psychiatrist prior to the first session.

When the therapist contacted the psychiatrist, he informed the doctor of the family history and the course of treatment. The psychiatrist assessed David and said he believed that David should be started on a trial of medication for ADHD. The school reported immediate improvement.

Follow-up

The therapist called the family one month later. Katherine reported that the family meetings were being continued and that the children were doing well and behaving much better. She stated that the medication had helped David to concentrate and stay focused on tasks in school. In addition, she stated that she had been feeling better and had not used laxatives since her first visit to the PCP. She said that she felt more secure in her relationship with her husband, and that as the family learned to communicate, all of their relationships improved. When the therapist asked if Katherine felt that the family needed further sessions, she replied that they did not at this time, but would continue with David's psychiatrist. The therapist explained that if they were ever in need of therapy, Katherine should contact the MCO for authorization. Finally, the therapist sent a termination summary to the MCO closing the case.

What Went Right

The therapist, working from a strategic family therapy perspective, assessed that the problem did not lie solely within the children. Instead, there was a focus on the interactional patterns of the family. The therapist communicated with the MCO case manager when the assessment could not be completed in one session, and kept the lines of communication open as the treatment plan changed. The therapist designed the interventions to take place at home, which allowed the therapist to fine-tune the interaction while the family was in the therapy room. In addition, this allowed the family to make changes in a briefer period of time. Finally, the therapist coordinated the care with the other professionals involved, which greatly helped the course of treatment to flow.

THE STRUCTURAL APPROACH

An interview with a family therapist* who works for a national managed care company explained how structural fam-

---

*Nadine Mackintosh, Ph.D., LMFT, is a salaried therapist and case manager at MCC Behavioral Care, Inc, in South Florida. Dr. Mackintosh holds a doctorate in family therapy.

ily therapy (Minuchin & Fishman, 1981) is easily applied to the work done under managed care especially when adolescents are involved. Similar to strategic family therapy, structural family therapy is generally characterized as working to reorganize dysfunctional hierarchies by putting the parents in charge of the children and differentiating among subsystems within families (Madanes & Haley, 1977).

Structural family therapy is an active, problem-solving approach to a dysfunctional family context (Minuchin & Fishman, 1981). Salvador Minuchin (1974), the major proponent of structural family therapy, points out that this therapy is characterized by its emphasis on hierarchical issues. Correcting the dysfunctional family hierarchies and making strong differentiations among the subsystems of the family are generally achieved by modifying the way people relate to one another. Minuchin (1974) states that the therapy is complete when the family can adapt to the new hierarchies and maintain itself without the use of the presenting problem.

Putting this theory in pragmatic terms, Mackintosh (personal communication, 1995) describes the course of therapy with adolescents following a basic step model. The first step is for the therapist to investigate communication patterns within the family. The family generally uses the presenting problem to sustain unhealthy communication and alliances (Minuchin, 1974). Therefore, the second step is to study the family alliances. It is often common for one of the children in the family to align with one of the parents, which can lead to triangulation within the family (Minuchin, 1974). The third step is to understand the reasons for the triangulation that is taking place in the family. The next step would be for the therapist to gain an understanding of the reasons behind any scapegoating that takes place in the family. Finally, the therapist gets ready to move the family forward by looking for family/individual strengths on which to start building independence and planning for termination (Mackintosh, personal communication, 1995).

The goal of therapy can be diagrammed in the following way.

Move the family from:

$$\frac{\text{Child}}{\text{Mother/Father}} \quad \text{to} \quad \frac{\text{Mother/Father}}{\text{Child}}$$

In a managed care environment where clients have a limited number of benefits for a calendar year, it is important for the therapist to be cognizant of using benefits wisely. Since the emphasis is on immediate in-session behaviors and the therapist generally works with the entire family, structural family therapy should start with weekly sessions until the presenting problem is stabilized; then move to every other week for two to three sessions. Finally, the sessions should move to monthly for one to two months to maintain stabilization. This brings the average length of total sessions to within the five to nine session range.

CASE EXAMPLES

The Kid Who Wanted Out

Candace came to therapy with her mother because she had been truant from school. This was not a new behavior for Candace, as she had a history of psychiatric treatment for depression, attention-deficit disorder, and oppositional defiant disorder and other therapy treatments. The mother had been raising Candace alone as the father was in jail for murder. Mother felt that her daughter was out of control and that she was unable to be effectual in her parenting.

When Candace and her mother came into therapy, the family setup could have been described in this way:

Candace (Father
_____
Mother

It was evident that Candace was in control of the home and her mother. In order to avoid conflict her mother would not speak up. Her father was physically peripheral as he was in jail; however, Candace was aligned with him or, at least, the fantasy of him. In many ways, Candace would ask for her mother to be in control. She would do this by acting out. However, each time Candace would act out, her mother would simply remain quiet. In turn, Candace would escalate her next action in the hope that her mother would react. Her mother would finally respond when an outside agency became involved, and she would then bring Candace to therapy. This time, the therapy began only a few months prior to the father's release from prison.

From the first session, the therapist brought the father into the therapy by using an empty chair and involving his "voice" in the questions. It became apparent to the therapist that Candace was being loyal to him during the sessions as she would escape from the questions and responsibility by not answering. The therapist saw this as being isomorphic to Dad's past escape from prison.

The mother was also loyal, as she had remained married to him for his entire prison stay. She helped Candace maintain her relationship with her father by bringing her to weekend visits at the state penitentiary. In addition, the mother welcomed the idea of renewing a marital relationship with her husband.

The goal of the therapy was to realign the hierarchies in the family and strengthen the subsystems. When the therapy is completed, the family should have the parents parenting Candace in a mutually agreeable fashion no matter what the state of their marital relationship is. The final picture should look like this:

Mother/Father
_____
Candace

When the therapy began, the therapist noted that Candace was attempting to manipulate the parental relationship since the father would soon be released. Outside of the familial relationship, Candace was having relationship problems with boys. She had been acting out in ways that were inappropriate for her age of 14 years. When asked why they had come to therapy, the mother stated that she was concerned that Candace's behavior was going to get her into real trouble, and Candace reported that she was concerned about her mother's depression.

The therapist decided to introduce the father's voice in order to help the mother and Candace move from their stuck position. The therapist asked about what the father would need to do in order to be successful upon his release. Candace said that he would need to learn to follow rules as well as how to deal with stress. The therapist pursued this line of thought and asked Candace if she thought her dad was going to be able to manage or would he wind up back in prison. Candace thought her dad could succeed if he really put his mind to it, and said she believed he would. She added that she felt that she and her mother needed to get their acts together. When asked what this meant, Candace replied that she felt that her mother needed to get back on antidepressants and that she herself needed to start watching her behavior and to go back to school.

The therapist spoke with the mother about the need to put her own life in order before she would be able to help her daughter. The mother agreed to see the psychiatrist and to make sure that Candace went back to school. She did see the psychiatrist, but it was evident that the changes occurring with Candace were self-motivated. Candace was attending school regularly, she had stopped acting out sexually, her talk was more age-appropriate, and she was showing appropriate affect instead of her previous tough exterior.

The family was now in a position where the father was higher than Candace and the mother was peripheral. The family looked like this:

Father (Mother

Candace

The therapist filed a treatment summary that stated the goals achieved to date: the goal to decrease behavioral outbursts had been reached, as evidenced by Candace's changes in deportment. An unachieved goal was to create an appropriate parental relationship, one that sanctioned the parents being in charge of their child. The current stage of therapy spoke to maintaining the goals already achieved until the father was released from prison. He had been made aware of the therapy process by Candace, and an invitation has been extended to him to attend sessions upon his return. At that time, the therapist would be able to ascertain whether he was a customer for change. If he was willing to participate, then the course of therapy would be set to achieve the goal of parental repositioning. If Dad was unwilling to be part of the therapy, then the goal would have to be restructured to include the mother and Candace only.

What Went Right

In this case, the therapist worked for the MCO and had the dual role of therapist and case manager. Keeping the benefit limit purchased by the mother's employer in mind, the therapist had to remember that there was a time limit to therapy based on these benefits. Therefore, the therapist frequently staffed the case with the psychiatrist and alternated sessions so that they did not overlap. And, since as the family was in limbo until the father was released, the sessions were more spread out in order to keep the mother and daughter in a maintenance mode.

We Just Wanted to Be Her Friend

The MCO intake department was contacted by a father who stated that he and his wife had been disagreeing on how to parent their daughter. He stated that his daughter was breaking her curfew, hanging out with strange people, and being defiant of the house rules. The father requested a referral to a therapist.

The parents attended the first session without their daughter (Andrea). They reported that when they told Andrea where they were going, she did not return home from school. The mother was visibly upset. When asked by the therapist why she was so upset, she reported that the couple had waited so long to have a child, and they hoped that, as she grew up, they would be close friends and be able to respect one another. She was upset because she did not believe that their daughter respected them.

The therapist spent most of the session explaining that they needed to be the parents, especially during the tumultuous adolescent years. They needed to set rules for Andrea and establish what the consequences would be if these rules were broken. The therapist also talked to them about how to get Andrea to come to the next session.

The treatment plan was submitted to the MCO case manager with the primary focus on the parents. The goals of therapy were to achieve a strong parental subsystem, to realign the subsystems so that the parents were in charge of their child, and to help the parents to set rules and devise consequences for breaking those rules.

The therapist reported that Andrea did attend the second session, and the therapist asked the parents how they were able to get her to do so. They said that they simply told her that she had to come with them. They stated that they did not give her a choice. Andrea was somewhat apprehensive about going to counseling.

Now, with Andrea present, the therapist asked the mother and father what they believed the problem to be. They again repeated that they were concerned that Andrea was not obeying their rules and they were very upset by this. Andrea replied by asking what rules they had set. She looked at the therapist and stated that she was not given rules, and that her parents seemed to make things up as they went along. The therapist asked the parents to explain what types of rules they would like to have in their home. They talked first about a curfew. As the discussion progressed, it became evident to the therapist that the parents could not agree on a curfew between themselves. In addition, they wanted to set different curfews for different occasions, for example, Saturday night with a party, Saturday night with a date, Saturday night with friends.

The therapist explored what happened in the family when Andrea did not obey the curfew. The parents described a situation in which it was shown that the parents would fight because the father would want to punish Andrea for breaking curfew, whereas the mother would want to talk with Andrea about the evening she had experienced. Inevitably, the parents would fight, Andrea would go to bed, and no one would address the rules or set consequences for Andrea.

The therapist submitted a treatment update that had the primary goal of the parents being able to set mutually agreeable rules and consequences for breaking the rules. The therapist expressed that the way this would be achieved was through direct conversation during the sessions, which would help the parents to understand the control that they allowed Andrea to have over them. Through these interventions, the therapist's secondary goal was to realign the subsystems and strengthen the couple's relationship.

The therapist submitted a termination summary to the MCO case manager only eight sessions later. The termination summary showed that the total number of sessions was ten. At first, the therapist met with the family weekly. This continued for six sessions. During this time, the therapist helped to reveal to the parents how they had let Andrea run the house and to make clear that at 15 years of age, she was not capable of running herself, let alone the entire family. The therapist also educated the mother to the fact that it was not appropriate for her to be Andrea's friend and to give up on parenting. The therapist explained that there needed to be a balance. Once the subsystems were realigned, the therapist moved the sessions to every other week and then monthly. The total course of treatment was three months. The prognosis was good and the therapy ended because all the treatment goals were met.

What Went Right

The therapist had a well-documented course of treatment. Although it is not necessary to spell out the theory with which

you are working, in this case it helped the case manager to understand clearly the treatment goals and the course of treatment. The therapist completed the paperwork in a timely manner so that care could be authorized and deemed appropriate. Finally, the therapist ended therapy with a good prognosis based on the resolution of the problem.

MCOs are looking more and more to therapists to not just patch up a situation, but to find solutions to problems so that the client acquires the skills to apply to similar problems as well. The reason for this is twofold. First, it is clinically and ethically important for clients to find symptom relief and to be able to walk away from the therapy experience with skills that help them to be better prepared to solve problems on their own. Second, when the problem is addressed correctly the first time and the client has skills to apply to other situations, the client is less likely to represent to treatment. This is a financially sound prospect to the MCOs, which are generally providing benefits under the assumption that only a certain percentage of covered individuals will present for treatment.

THE MILAN APPROACH

The Milan approach to family therapy (Selvini Palazzoli et al., 1978) shares similar beliefs with the MRI group and the Haley/Madanes version of strategic family therapy in that they all view problems as being maintained by behavioral sequences. These tenets were founded and influenced by the early work of Gregory Bateson (Piercy & Sprenkle, 1986). However, MRI therapy and strategic family therapy were additionally influenced by the work of Milton H. Erickson, whereas the Milan group held true to Bateson's original works. One of the most basic differences between these two schools of thought is the level at which change occurs. In both the MRI approach and strategic family therapy, change occurs behaviorally first, which affects the client's beliefs about the problems. However, the Milan approach believes that change first occurs on the semantic level, which affects the client's behavior.

The therapists of the Milan Group (Selvini Palazzoli, Boscolo, Cecchin, & Prata, 1978) learned that a successful intervention is the therapy session itself. They designed the therapy session to be structured to have the most impact on the family's semantics of the problem, which would in turn have an impact on the family's behavior (Selvini Palazzoli, Boscolo, Cecchin, & Prata, 1980). As seen in the aforementioned family therapies, the therapist takes responsibility for creating the change within the family or client system. This is done through observing the interactions and creating direct or indirect interventions. Tomm (1984) explains that the Milan Group uses the session as the intervention because of its belief that the family is ever-changing, but that problems are created when the client's beliefs do not fit the current pattern of behaviors.

Through the session interventions of hypothesizing, remaining neutral, and the use of circular questioning (Selvini Palazzoli et al., 1980), the therapist creates an environment in which the family can start to adopt new understandings and beliefs, which in turn causes behavioral changes.

The Milan Group designed a course of questioning known as circular questioning (Selvini Palazzoli et al., 1980), which allows for information to surface in ways that it had not previously. The therapists hypothesize about what they believe the family's problem to be. The therapist asks questions that involve all participants (present or not) based on these hypotheses. The questioning allows the therapist and the family to continue to rework the hypotheses until they mutually create one that allows the family to begin to create change. The circularity is exhibited in the way in which the therapist asks one family member to comment on the inter-actional patterns of others (Penn, 1982). This allows the family members to view their own behaviors and the behaviors of others in a context that they may not have seen before. This new context alone may foster change.

Different from the work of structural family therapists, therapists using the Milan approach remain neutral and avoid issues of hierarchy. The therapist actually maintains partiality to all members of the system in order to preserve maneuverability within the system. This neutrality allows family members to choose whether or not to change, which is aligned with the goal of simply exposing the family to a new way of viewing their problem. In cases where the therapist needs to be sensitive to the length of treatment, as well as in all therapy where family therapy is the prime modality, circular questioning allows the therapist to gather a lot of pertinent information in a short time. In addition, the therapist often sees that the information that evolves guides clients to generate their own out-of-session interventions.

CASE EXAMPLES

They Are Kicking Her Out of Day Care

A family therapist who works for a national managed care organization* was called in for a consult when a therapist was facing a stuck case. The client's 4-year-old daughter had been kicked out of day care, and the mother had brought "her

---

*Betty Davis, Ph.D., LMFT, is a salaried employee of MCC Behavioral Care in South Florida. Dr. Davis is the Clinical Administrator of MCC's Behavioral Care Offices. She holds a doctorate degree in family therapy.

little monster" to therapy at the request of the intake specialist because she wanted the child to go to an inpatient setting for care. During the first session, the mother and the therapist became involved in a verbal battle because the therapist tried to explain to the mother that inpatient care was not medically necessary and that it would not achieve a longterm goal. Each time the therapist tried to point out that hospitalization is reserved for rapid stabilization when individuals are in danger of hurting themselves or others, the mother would escalate the discussion. Finally, the therapist called in the consultant, who took a more circular approach.

The consultant knew it would be futile to continue the positive escalation because the mother was not a customer for education. In all reality, the mother was looking to use her inpatient benefits to find day care. Circular questions allowed the consultant and the mother to engage in a factfinding conversation. This then allowed the therapy conversation to be the intervention and the process to move along.

The consultant began by asking the mother why she was coming to therapy and what she hoped to get out of it. She reiterated that she wanted to put her child in an inpatient setting. The consultant began to ask questions that were not in direct response to the statement, but that started to reveal information about how all the individuals involved felt about the situation. The questions revealed that the child had been in a children's shelter when the mother was unable to care for her. In that surrounding, chaos makes sense. In addition, it came out that the stepfather was unable to cope with the energy level of the child and refused to believe it was his problem and so would not come to therapy. In addition, the stepfather was concerned about what kind of influence his stepdaughter would have on the new baby in the family—his biological child. The mother was asked to describe what influence, if any, she thought the new baby had on her daughter's behavior.

After all the information was gathered, the consultant

stated that the problem did not seem to really lie within the child, but in the family and the context of her short and chaotic life. The mother then restated the problem as her need to put her daughter away because her husband did not understand the girl's behavior. He was actually afraid of her behavior. This put the mother in an awkward position as she felt that the only way to keep her daughter under control was constantly to yell and try to stifle her child's 4-year-old behavior.

The mother was then able to see that her request was one that could not be fulfilled. She admitted to feeling trapped and wanting to keep the stepfather happy as she had another child to think about. She realized herself that her 4-year-old was simply acting her age. When questioned about the way the day care personnel thought about her child's behavior, the mother reported that the daughter had been kicked out of two day care centers because she was not "controllable."

After considerable conversation, the consultant was able to back the mother away from her original request. At that time, the mother stated that she was willing to explore other options. She agreed to have an evaluation with the psychiatrist to see if medications would be appropriate for her daughter. In order to avoid false hopes, she was warned that medication would not be magic. She was counseled that the ideal situation would be for everyone to come to family therapy to work on their differences and to educate the parents to better parenting skills.

What Went Right

Clients may leave the process without getting exactly what they came for. Sometimes, as in this case, what the client wants is not considered medically necessary by the MCO. The most important thing to remember is not to triangulate the client and MCO just because the client asks for a particular service. Sometimes a little bit of education goes a long way. Some clients will recalibrate and look for alternative solutions, whereas others will continue to escalate. This is a phenomenon that HMOs are used to as many clients are still not comfortable with a managed product. The MCO will expect you to work to educate the client as best you can, and when all else fails to refer the client to the MCO case manager or customer service department. The most important thing you as the therapist can do in this case is to contact the MCO case manager and inform him or her of the situation so that what you explained to the client is clear to the case manager.

Tell My Mother I Am Not Gay

Jason came to the initial session after being referred by the MCO intake coordinator. He stated that he wanted to find a way to help his parents understand that he was not homosexual. Doing work for an MCO often means that the therapist may change some of the normal work routines. Therefore, the therapist had Jason come to the office early to do the paperwork. The therapist then conducted the first session as a psychosocial assessment to fulfill the requirements of the MCO. The therapist, who had worked with this MCO for a number of years, was well aware of what information was requested on the initial review. Most of the first session was spent gathering information on the client's medical history, previous psychotherapeutic treatment, current and past medication, current and past substance abuse, and so on. Finally, the therapist asked Jason what he interpreted his problem to be.

During the telephone review of the treatment plan, the therapist explained that Jason stated that he had been involved in a homosexual relationship in the past, but that he believed that at the present time he was ready to commit to a heterosexual relationship. His reported reason for this was that he wanted to get married and have a family of his own. Jason reported that he felt that people assumed he was homosexual and were having difficulty understanding his new choices. The therapist explained to the case manager that he questioned Jason about who else believed that he was not homosexual. Jason stated to the therapist that his friends believed him, as did a woman with whom he had just entered into a relationship. When asked who was the most likely not to believe him, he stated that it would be his parents, especially his mother.

The therapist reported that he continued to use circular questions to understand the client's interpretation of the problem. The therapist reported that Jason felt that he had devastated his mother two years earlier when he announced his involvement in a homosexual relationship. He said that although his family was very supportive of his lifestyle, he felt that at that time his mother's dream of grandchildren had died. He was convinced that his mother believed that an individual could not choose whether or not to be homosexual. He was concerned that she would not believe in his choice and that there would always be doubt between them.

Finally, the therapist reported that he had planned to move forward by bringing Jason's family together for a family session. He had worked with Jason to design the session, educating Jason to the idea that he might not be able to convince his mother, but that opening a discussion would be a good start.

The therapist contacted the case manager not more than two weeks later to state that he was closing the case. He reported that the family session had taken place one week earlier. When Jason appeared for the session, he reported to the therapist that he had already started the discussion at home.

He remembered what the therapist told him and accepted his mother's skepticism. This had an unusual effect on his mother.

During the family session, the mother explained to the therapist that at first she was very skeptical that her son could change his lifestyle. She stated that as Jason took a watch and see attitude, she started to believe that it might be true. The mother reportedly asked the therapist if he believed that Jason could now be heterosexual. The therapist remained neutral and stated that it did not matter what he believed—what counted was what Jason believed and how Jason chose to live his life. In addition, the therapist explained to the mother that he could understand her skepticism and asked her questions about how she could maintain her skepticism and still leave room to change her mind. The therapist explained that he had asked both the father and Jason what the mother's doubt meant. He also asked the father to explain how he saws his wife's skepticism affecting Jason.

The therapist reported that the family was content with the family session and did not choose to schedule a second visit. One week later, the therapist contacted Jason to follow up. Jason stated that he was very happy because he had found a way to express himself to his mother and had learned that it was not truly important what she believed, but more important that she accepted him and his choices. Jason felt that he did not need any additional services. The therapist reported that the stated treatment goals had been met and the prognosis was fair. He told Jason to contact the MCO should he need services in the future.

What Went Right

The therapist gained an understanding of the client's belief system. In addition, the therapist understood that the changes would be more semantic than behavioral. The therapist hypothesized that the client wanted his mother to change her beliefs, which was too great a task for the therapy to undertake. Once this was discussed, the therapist, through the use of circular questions, helped the client to develop clear and attainable goals for the therapy and for the family. Finally, the therapist clearly documented the reason for such brief treatment. With a follow-up phone call, the therapist had documented a reason for closure. The sessions acted as the interventions, moving Jason and his mother from their fixed positions to a place where they were both able to accept that change might be possible.

SUMMARY

As can be seen by the preceeding case examples, strategic therapies allow great flexibility for therapists as well as for clients. This flexibility helps the therapist to introduce changes that provide results in fewer sessions. The future trend of benefits packages looks like the number of annual sessions will decrease from the already low numbers. Given these restrictions, therapists need to promote change in an effective manner that does not burden the client more (i.e., financially). Strategic therapies allow for change with limited intrusion. Finally, success with modalities highlighted in this chapter, as well as in the previous one, will strengthen relationships with MCOs. Therapists can then focus on serving many happy clients in a shorter time as opposed to one or two clients for a long time.

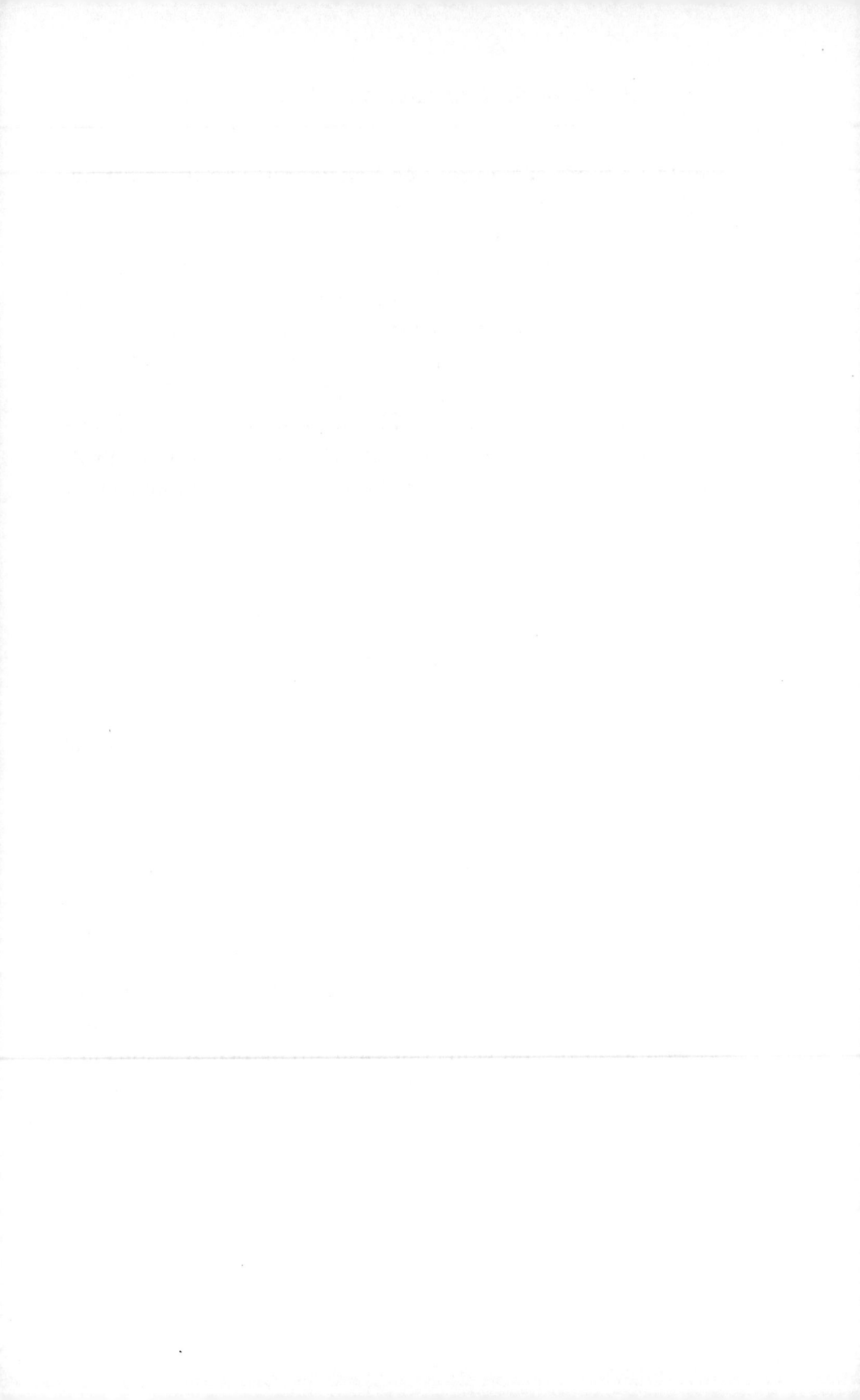

6

Case Management

As therapists, we can see how cases make sense from a clinical perspective. The MCO's case managers are generally licensed clinicians or nurses. They have administrative training added to their formal therapeutic education and clinical experience. The MCO's case managers must carefully balance both clinical and administrative perspectives in managing their cases. This chapter provides case scenarios that show the therapist how to describe treatment plans in behavioral terms so that they make sense to case managers. In addition, the chapter focuses on how to update these treatment plans as the care progresses so that the therapist learns to use the appropriate language to justify the continuation of authorization of care. The key to this stage is clarifying the medical for necessity of care and a spirit of a collaborative partnership with the MCO.

Finally, the importance of the case management skills in order to be successful in the arena of managed care is explained. There are many different professionals that therapists may need to consult in order to maintain a systemic spin to their therapy. Possibly one of the most difficult tasks is to manage a case and coordinate information among professionals.

WEARING THE LENS OF THE CASE MANAGER

The term "medical necessity" is often one that is difficult to define in the field of mental health. Its common connotation is "medically appropriate." For example, in outpatient cases when clear behavioral goals can be set and met, the care might considered medically appropriate. However, if behavioral goals cannot be set and the care is taking on a supportive or hand-holding tone, then the care is not medically appropriate.

Since these distinctions can be difficult to define, the following case scenario will explain the difference between what is medically appropriate and what is not.

See It Through an Example

Samantha,* a 35-year-old woman, is married and has two daughters, ages 4 and 6 years. Samantha's mother also lives

---

*All names have been changed in order to maintain confidentiality.

in the house with the family. The family lives in a small town with limited mental health resources. Samantha's husband is a factory worker who makes barely enough money to support the family. He is the insurance subscriber.

The couple has had marital problems dating back to the beginning of their marriage. Each time the couple has a fight, Samantha becomes "suicidal." She has been known to cut her wrists, but never cuts deep enough to cause major damage, although her wrists have been stitched up numerous times. All family members are aware of this, and the children have learned to mimic their mother. The younger child, while playing at a friend's house, put red paint on her wrists and stated that she was acting like her mother. Samantha's mother thought she was helping by telling her daughter how to be a better mother and wife. Neither Samantha nor her mother work outside the home.

Samantha had one other problem that was uncovered during her first hospitalization; she grew her own marijuana and had used it daily for the previous five years. Samantha was hospitalized for rapid stabilization after she slit her wrists, and remained in the hospital for three weeks. Each time the doctor discussed discharge Samantha said she was suicidal. Finally, a therapist was brought in to meet with Samantha to create a bridge to outpatient care.

This incident happened at the beginning of a benefit year. Samantha had a total of 30 inpatient days for the calendar year, and now 21 days had been used. Given the severity of her crisis, the goal for therapy was to engage the family in treatment and find appropriate coping strategies so that Samantha would not have to escalate to the point of hospitalization. The client/family had 30 outpatient visits for mental health and 30 outpatient visits for substance abuse in a calendar year.

What Went Wrong

The therapist continued building a bridge with the client and her family and sent in a treatment plan that outlined a course of individual therapy that focused on getting Samantha in touch with her anger with her mother. The therapy goals were to decrease anger by finding its root, to help the client to gain autonomy from her family of origin by having her keep a journal, and to help the client to get ready for family therapy. The estimated number of sessions was 12.

Let us look at why the case manager would find this an ineffective treatment plan. First, the therapist has proposed to use 12 of the 30 sessions to "get the client ready" for family work. Given that the client lived with her family, it was too much to hope that the dysfunctional interactional patterns could be put on hold until the client was ready to deal with them. Second, the goal of helping the client to gain autonomy from her family of origin was too great a goal given that Samantha's mother lived in the same house. The goals were not spelled out in behavioral terms and therefore were not measurable. Neither the therapist nor the client would be able to measure success. In addition, the client could have been set up for failure in that she might never "be ready for family therapy." Last, the therapist described this treatment plan to Samantha despite the verbalized concern by the MCO's case manager. This step then triangulated the client, therapist, and MCO.

When the therapist tried to explain a change in treatment plan as suggested by the case manager, Samantha became angry and called the MCO case manager. She told the case manager that if the treatment plan was changed, she would kill herself. Given that the ultimate goal was to keep the client safe and try to avoid another hospitalization, the case manager agreed to authorize the individual therapy for the 12 sessions.

The client quickly became dependent on the therapist, calling at all hours of the night and day. At the end of the 12th session, the therapist tried to bring the family in for family therapy. By this time, the family felt relief from Samantha since she now burdened the therapist with all of her concerns. Therefore, the family was very reluctant to come to therapy. Samantha often called to request individual therapy for each of her family members.

The therapist used all of Samantha's outpatient mental health sessions very quickly, making very little progress in helping the client to identify appropriate coping strategies and coping mechanisms for herself. The therapist agreed to see Samantha on a sliding fee scale, but the client refused because she did not believe that she should pay for services. Since the family was not engaged successfully in treatment, the sessions could not be authorized under the husband's benefits because he would not be attending. The children's benefits were disallowed because the therapist did not make a philosophical bridge for Samantha. Samantha could not see that her problems affected her children and she would not bring them for conjoint sessions. Samantha's therapy ended, and approximately two months later, she called the MCO and told the case manager that she was going to slit her wrists. The police were contacted and Samantha was re-admitted to an inpatient psychiatric unit for stabilization. This time Samantha only had nine inpatient days left.

What Went Right

Samantha called the MCO when her new benefit year began. She stated that she was suicidal and the case manager tried to get Samantha to contract for her safety, but when all efforts failed she was immediately hospitalized for rapid stabilization. This time her hospital stay lasted for a full 30 days; as before, each time her discharge was planned, she stated that she was suicidal.

During her hospital stay, a new family therapist was brought to meet Samantha. The therapist was informed of Samantha's history and quickly put a plan in place to have the family come in for treatment while she was still in the hospital. The therapist enlisted the help of the psychiatrist, who called the family members and told them that it was imperative for them to come for treatment. They agreed.

When Samantha was released from the hospital, the therapist had the entire family in for a treatment planning session. During this session, the therapist explained who would need to come into the sessions, when they would need to come in, and who would need to go with Samantha to see the psychiatrist. The therapist also discussed a plan to enroll Samantha in a substance abuse treatment program and/or self-help group. The family and Samantha agreed to the treatment plan. Samantha started to make progress. She and her husband started to work on their marital problems. Samantha's mother agreed to consider moving out of the house and Samantha started to look for a job.

Update

Samantha continues to have problems within her family. She has remained drug-free for one year, but when things get stressful, she still threatens to hurt herself. However, she maintains a good relationship with the therapist since the therapist has stretched the time between sessions so that Samantha is not left without covered sessions. The therapist always includes the medical necessity for treatment on her treatment updates. In addition, she introduced Samantha to the community mental health center in case inpatient services are needed in the future. The therapist interfaces with the psychiatrist to assure better treatment and Samantha has not needed to become an inpatient even when faced with the life stressor of her mother's death. Samantha's newly found coping strategies worked through a very stressful time—she did not relapse.

The case manager would be looking at the medical necessity of ongoing care. In a particularly difficult case such as Samantha's, the case manager would want to see how continued outpatient treatment could help to avoid another inpatient stay. Even in the case where a client uses all the inpatient days available for one year, helping to keep the client out of the hospital rings favorably because it can be argued that the client has learned more appropriate coping strategies.

SUMMARY

Remember, no matter how difficult or how simple the case, always keep in mind the perspective of the MCO while planning treatment. Many therapists state that this is what makes them feel that they have given up their autonomy when working with the MCO. However, the "What Went Right" outlined course of therapy is focused, has behaviorally measured goals, and creates the difference that makes a difference, no matter what theoretical approach is applied to the actual therapy done in the confines of the clinician's office.

Finding an appropriate way to talk about, explain, or exemplify the good treatment you provide should not be a hindrance, but a necessity. Understanding the language of managed care and using it when speaking with the MCO case managers help to promote a spirit of partnership. This is no different than joining the world view of your clients (Haley, 1985). Always describe your work in a way that shows off its clinical-effectiveness, cost-effectiveness, and time-sensitivity.

Speaking to Other Professionals

Many therapists fall into the trap of a false sense of security or knowledge that they "own a case." Often the professional does not speak to other professionals involved and they try to work in a vacuum. This can lead to many problems. Family therapists have long learned how to coordinate care in order to work from the most educated position when starting a case.

Interfacing with Case Managers

Often therapists are on various provider panels and learn to work differently from MCO to MCO. More frequently than not, the provider may not know what to expect when getting involved in the care review process. Providers often feel as though they are put on the spot to defend their work. Sometimes the most disparaging part of the process is to find that MCOs do not provide care management that is isomorphic to the solution-oriented approach that they ask their providers to work from. Current trends show that this will change, but until that time, solution-oriented, time-sensitive therapists may find that they spend more time explaining things to the case managers than they spend on therapy with their clients.

I Called, But No One Was Home

Working in an environment where care is being reviewed for authorization allows this author to hear reactions from providers about the care management process. Some processes move more easily than others. One family therapist who studied extensively with the Brief Family Therapy Center in Milwaukee telephoned to do a clinical review for ongoing cases. The case manager was only vaguely familiar with solution-focused therapy. The therapist began to explain the family's story. The following conversation took place.

Therapist: The family came in because the son was having a lot of trouble in school. This 8-year-old boy just started to run away from the bus stop each morning when his father dropped him off.

Case Mgr.: Uh huh. What is the diagnosis?

Therapist: Well, it really seems to be a problem with the family because he started to act this way when he heard his parents fight and threaten to get divorced. The son then stated that he was afraid to go to school.

Case Mgr.: So, you are diagnosing a school phobia for the child?

Therapist: No, because the boy really likes school. He just doesn't want to leave his parents alone because he is afraid that they will fight if he is not around. I diagnosed this as a parent–child problem.

Case Mgr.: Okay, so what is the treatment plan?

Therapist: I will see the family together to work on solutions to the problem. Actually, they already have solutions, but they just don't realize it. We will work on finding the solutions that already are in place and help them to build on their success. The couple already understands how their relationship has an impact on their son and have stopped fighting in front of him. I would say that between the time they first called for therapy and now, they have made approximately a 50% improvement. Our goals are to decrease the fighting in front of the son, to help the son to understand that the couple's problems do not reflect negatively on their love for him, and to decrease the running away from the school bus stop, which means school attendance will improve.

Case Mgr.: Don't you think that you will need to spend time alone with the son?

Therapist: No. This is an interactional problem, not a problem that lies solely in the son. I *am* working from a solution-focused model. I think four to five sessions will be all that I need to wrap this case up.

Case Mgr.: Are you sure that we do not need to register the parents separately so that they can get marital counseling? And I am concerned because when they first called in they stated that the problem was with their child. Now, it sounds like you are diagnosing the family and not the son.

Therapist: I do not think it is necessary to split up the family's care when it can all be handled with one therapist in a short period of time. The idea here is to be the least intrusive possible.

The therapist became increasingly frustrated. He contacted the supervisor of the case manager and decribed the conversation. He told the supervisor that he knew someone was on the other end of the phone, but he felt that "no one was home." The therapist explained that the MCO expected the therapists to work from a solution-oriented approach, but it did not seem as though the case managers employed by the MCOs were well versed in such approaches.

This type of experience has led recent research* to take a provider's look at managed care case management. One hundred managed mental health care providers were surveyed about care management practices. The research took a unique focus as the researcher (Earhart, personal communication, 1995) asked the managed care providers to state what questions they would expect a managed care case manager to ask if the case manager were working from a solution-oriented approach.

Managed care companies cannot survive without solid and mature provider panels that are willing to partner with the company. As the industry demand for more quality at lower costs increases, the MCOs look for new ways to partner with the providers (i.e., shared financial risk programs). Until this time, the demands have been initiated by the MCOs and thrust upon the providers.

To step outside of the box and remain systemic, the MCOs must see that that the relationship needs to be collaborative. The MCOs need to ask themselves what they should do differently so that the providers feel a greater commitment, trust, and partnership. As in any relationship, the best way to find out what the other partner feels is to ask. This simple concept often seems foreign in the world of big business.

---

*Michael Earhart is a Clinical Team Leader for MCC Behavioral Care's National Service Center located in Eden Prairie, Minnesota. Michael is currently working on his PsyD at the University of St. Thomas in Minnesota, where his primary research is on solution-oriented care management.

Accordingly, Earhart (personal communication, 1995) showed that the providers who are truly working from a solution-oriented perspective will expect MCO professionals to work from the same perspective. The following is an aggregate list of questions that the surveyed providers would expect the MCOs to ask* if the MCO were working from a solution-oriented approach.

- Why has the client come to therapy now?
- Has some life-cycle event/change, anniversary reaction, status change, crisis, or outside event affected the client's decision to come in at this time?
- Why now as opposed to some weeks ago or some weeks from now?
- Whose idea was it that the client come in? What is his/her hope and concern for the client? What does the client think/feel about this?

What are the presenting problems/symptoms?

- What does the client say is going on?
- What would he/she like to change by seeing you?

What is the current impact of the problem/symptoms?

- On a scale of 1 to 10, with 10 being the most severe problem the client could have and 1 being the least, how does the client rate the current problem?

What is the client's level of motivation?

- On a scale of 1 to 10, with 10 correlating with the client being willing to do anything he/she can to solve the problem and 1 correlating with the clients not

*This information has been reproduced with the permission of the researcher, Michael Earhart.

being willing to do anything about it, how does the client rate his/her motivation?

How will the client know it is time to stop coming to see you?

- How will the client know when his/her therapy is sufficient?

- What will the client be doing differently when the issues that brought him/her to see you are less of a current problem?

What is your diagnostic assessment based on the client's clinical presentation (DSM-IV/Axes I–V)?
Does the client have any past mental health/substance abuse history?

- What therapy approaches have seemed to help in the past?

- What has the client done in the past to resolve these issues?

- If the client has relapsed in the past, what has helped him/her get back on track?

- What are the signs that he/she is on track?

Do you and/or the client assess the client to be at risk?

- How (to what degree, with what resources and support) has the client successfully dealt with or overcome being at risk in the past?

- How (to what degree, with what resources and support) is he/she successfully dealing with or overcoming being at risk now?

- What does the client say has kept him/her going (cope) when at risk in the past?

- What plan have you and the client formulated to overcome the current risk factors?

If medications have been part of past treatment approaches, what medications worked and what medications, if any, is the client taking or considering taking now?

What knowledge, strengths, and other resources does the client bring to this therapy?

- How can you and the client collaborate in ways that best use these resources?

- What does the client most respect about his/her own capacities that could help to surmount the current difficulties?

If a miracle were to occur and your client's concerns were resolved between sessions, what would be the first sign(s)?

- Who would be the first to notice?

- Who would not be surprised?

- Who would be among those most likely to celebrate the client's recovery?

- What is the client already doing that are signs of meeting his/her goals?

- How does this make a difference for the client?

What is the treatment plan for attaining the goals you and the client have identified and agreed to work on in therapy?

- What does the client think of this treatment plan?

- On a scale of 1 to 10 (with 1 being the farthest from and 10 being the closest to recovery), where does the client see himself/herself on the road to recovery?

- What would the client have to do to move one point up the scale?

How long does the client think it will take him/her to attain the goals?

- How many times does the client anticipate meeting with you in this time period?

- What does the client expect to do between sessions that will help him/her reach these goals?

It is not reasonable to believe that all of these questions would be asked in a review, especially if the information was provided to the MCO case manager in writing rather than by telephone. However, the questions do reflect the course of a thorough solution-oriented assessment. This research is ground-breaking because it can shape the managed care industry to be as responsible as the therapists providing the face-to-face care. If the case manager is sophisticated in solution-oriented treatment, this line of questioning allows the therapist to provide information to the case manager in a way similar to the manner in which the information was gathered from the client/client family. However, the potentially more valuable way in which this tool can be used is as a training tool.

Traditionally, the role of the MCO case manager has been to "scrutinize" the care of the provider and to determine whether or not the course of treatment deserves authorization. Currently, MCOs are moving toward the new generation of case management, which is more focused on network management than on case management. As therapists are analyzed to determine continued involvement on provider panels, the focus will be on practice patterns. As the case manager's role changes to take on a more educative/supervisory bent, the outlined course of questioning by Earhart (personal communication, 1995) will allow the more novice solution-oriented therapist to be exposed to the mind set. Case managers will act as supervisors to therapists who may not fully embrace the solution-oriented approaches. Selekman and Todd (1995) state that, "Even if the model is not fully adopted, the theoretical assumptions and techniques we [supervisors] present can provide new ways of establishing a cooperative climate" (p. 22).

The role of solution-oriented supervision has been reviewed (Marek, Sandifer, Beach, Coward, & Protinsky, 1994; Selekman & Todd, 1995; Todd and Selekman, 1991; Thomas, 1994; Welchler, 1990), and it has been shown that the supervisor and supervisee find the best results in learning when the two are working from the same model. This can easily be applied to the arena of managed care. This model would guide a more consultative approach to case management. As the case manager reviewed the case with the more sophisticated solution-oriented therapist, the focus of the questions could be on the therapist's view of the case and his or her role as the therapist (i.e., what tells you that you are on the right path with this client?).

Therapists do not stop practicing solution-oriented treatment after the initial assessment; therefore, solution-oriented MCO case management should not stop at the initial review. Such case management should continue through the concurrent review. In the continuation of the aforementioned research by Michael Earhart, therapists were asked what questions they expected to be asked during a solution-oriented concurrent review. The following are questions that providers felt a solution-oriented MCO case manager would ask.

On a scale of 1 to 10 (with 1 being the farthest away and 10 being the closest to recovery), where does the client now see him/herself on the road to recovery?

- What are the signs indicative of that change?

- What do you and the client see as having been the most helpful in moving up the path?

- What would the client have to do to move one point up the scale?

- How would he/she know that he/she got there?

What is the client's view of what has changed since the last review?

- What is the client doing that is helpful in reaching his/her goals?

- What are the clearest signs to the client that he/she is getting better?

- What knowledge, strengths, and other resources seem to be most helpful?

- What has the client been able to do differently now that he/she is finding solutions to problems?

Do you or the client identify any current risk factors?

- If yes, how are you collaborating to maximize the client's abilities to deal with or overcome them?

- If medications are a helpful part of the client's solution to his/her current problem, which ones prove most helpful and how does the client see the medication playing a role in his/her treatment goal?

Have you and the client made any changes in the treatment plan?

- How does the client feel about these changes and how they are going to help him/her reach the goals more effectively/more efficiently?

What does the client see happening over the next two to three months as he/she works on reaching the goals?

- How many times does the client expect to see you over that period?

- How does he/she see the therapy as helping him/her reach the goals?

- What does the client expect to be doing between sessions that will move him/her forward on the path?

What will tell the client that he/she is finished with this round of therapy?

- When does he/she expect this to happen?
- What will be the signs?
- What will you notice first?

What will the client be doing differently "living in the solution" than what he/she was doing when "under the influence of the problem"?

The simple assessment is that MCOs need to keep up with their provider panels, which have become more and more sophisticated in their clinical training and business strategies. As providers become better versed in solution-oriented approaches and need to utilize their time more cost-effectively, they will expect the MCO case managers to be equally knowledgeable so that clinical peer reviews run smoothly, based on a shared frame of reference and clearly identified expectations. The questions generated by this current research show that providers are capable of communicating about their therapeutic cases in ways that are appropriate to managed care.

As the case managers and providers become more sophisticated in this process, the role of each participant will probably change. One of the future trends for MCOs is to manage networks instead of the individual provider's clinical cases. This means that as providers have more time on the specific MCO panel, the understanding is that the case managers will have had ample opportunity to educate the provider about how the MCO works and how care is expected to be managed. This will then allow the providers to manage their own care and the case managers to review case histories retrospectively. With a retrospective review of provider's work (i.e., average length of stay by diagnosis, client satisfaction) the case managers will be able to focus on educating providers proactively. More than likely, as providers move toward this type of self-management status, the MCOs will have data-entry clerks entering the authorization for cases.

What Has Not Worked

Case managers need to have a complete and thorough understanding of the solution-oriented approaches to therapy; they also need to be financially focused and at the same time concentrate on the quality of services. In some instances, this has forced MCOs to develop continuous quality management and improvement programs. In these cases, MCOs have designed clinical programs and provider educational programs, and they follow documented level-of-care guidelines based on the therapeutic community's definition of best practices. Other companies are forced to deny care in order to maintain financial gains. When this happens, therapists become frustrated because communication with case managers can be difficult.

In one such case, the therapist contacted the case manager and stated the treatment plan outline along with behavioral goals. Without focusing on the clinical data provided, the case manager authorized 10 sessions. For some companies, the case managers do this as a standard routine. The therapist worked on the stated treatment goals with the client family, but the goals were not achieved within the 10 sessions because the situation was more acute than originally believed.

The therapist contacted the case manager to arrange for authorization of more sessions. The client's benefit package provided a total of 20 outpatient visits per calendar year. To date, only 11 sessions had been authorized. The therapist restated the clinical reasons why therapy should continue, outlining the severity of the problem, the lack of support that the identified patient felt within the family, the risk potential for hospitalization, and the fact that the original goals had not changed.

The case manager stated that he was unable to authorize additional sessions as the therapist had used the maximum number of sessions that he could authorize. The case manager informed the therapist that she would be receiving a denial-of-authorization letter in the mail. The therapist found herself in a difficult position in that she felt it would be clinically unethical to stop seeing the client. She understood that in addition to all of her other problems, the client had financial problems that would make it difficult for her to pay for services. The therapist did not want to triangulate the client and the MCO, which left her at a loss as to how to explain to the client that additional services were not authorized, especially when the therapist believed they were necessary.

The therapist once again tried to discuss the clinical data with the case manager, who finally suggested that the therapist file an appeal. With this, the therapist sent in the clinical records and waited for a decision on the appeal. In the meantime, the therapist continued to see the client, charging only the $10 copayment. The client started to show improvement. Each week, the therapist contacted the case manager to find out the status of the appeal. Finally, six weeks later, the therapist received a letter stating that the denial of authorization would be upheld.

This and similar situations have not been uncommon experiences for providers. The majority of managed care contracts have a legal clause that states that the provider may not charge the client for services that the MCO denies. The can put the provider in a compromising position when the provider feels that the care is medically necessary.

What Went Wrong

In this particular case, the case manager did not appear to be following a case review format that focuses on clinical care. The case manager did not find out if the client was a danger to self and/or others. The case manager did not negotiate alternative levels of care that would have allowed the client to find relief from the presenting problem while still fitting into the benefit package. Instead, the additional sessions were denied based on financial decisions. What some MCOs fail to realize is that providing the appropriate care at the right time, even if it means exhausting an individual's yearly benefits, can save money in the long run.

What Has Worked

MCOs that have learned to develop partnerships with their providers are best aligned to deliver quality clinical programs. In general, it seems that the MCOs that are treatment providers themselves have the most collaborative relationship with the panel providers. When the MCO and the provider maintain a true collaborative relationship, the communication is clear, and providers can make decisions in conjunction with the MCO case managers. This leads to better relationships from which clients also benefit in that all parties involved share a simple goal of quality care.

One of the biggest concerns for therapists is that they are clinically liable for a case even if the referral comes from the MCO. The providers want to know that their clinical impressions will hold weight with the MCOs. Providers who generally have the most success with this are those who have a clear understanding of the MCO's preferred practices. When the therapist can describe the care based on the preferred practices to which the MCO prescribes, the therapist then can justify the need for authorization of care.

Smooth Sailing

A client contacted her primary care physician to get a referral to see a therapist. The PCP asked the client to come in and see her. The PCP assessed that the client was anxious, wrote her a prescription for an antianxiety drug, and told the client to call back in one week to tell the PCP how she was doing.

The client called the PCP one week later. She explained that she still did not feel right and that she felt she needed to see a therapist. The PCP referred the client to see a therapist in her neighborhood, and contacted the case manager to inform him that the case was being turned over for concurrent review. In addition, the PCP contacted the therapist to tell him that this patient did not respond well to antianxiety medication.

The client (Marjorie) attended the first session and explained to the therapist that she was to be married in one month. Marjorie stated that she was very anxious about all the plans. She said that everyone was making demands on her and that she could not remember why she had agreed to have a wedding when she had originally wanted to elope. The therapist began to work with Marjorie to sort out the problem and to start to look at solutions. The therapist contacted the case manager in writing and stated that the goal of therapy was to help the client to understand where her anxiety was coming from and to involve her fiancé, and possibly her parents, in the therapy process. The therapy plan seemed simple.

As the therapy progressed, Marjorie began to reveal that

she was fearful of getting married because she was afraid that her fiancé would find out that she was bulimic. Once this came out into the open, Marjorie felt less anxious, especially when her fiancé stated that he understood and loved her no less. Therefore, the therapist continued to help the family find solutions to the wedding concerns so that Marjorie was not so overwhelmed by the pragmatic tasks.

The therapist sent in a treatment update form explaining the new diagnosis of bulimia. He also stated that he coordinated care with the primary care physician to make sure that Marjorie had no physical problems as a consequence of the bulimia. The therapist explained that the new goal was to get the bulimia under control, and to help the client establish healthier coping strategies to stressful situations, to find new ways to be in control of her emotions, and arrange a consultation appointment with a psychiatrist.

The case manager reviewing the treatment update forms believed that the course of treatment was accurate and arranged authorization for a consultation with a psychiatrist. The additional sessions were authorized. The therapist followed the outlined course of treatment and was able to measure progress in behavioral terms. However, when the 10 sessions were completed, the therapist felt that additional sessions were necessary. The therapist looked at the best practices for the treatment of bulimia. According to these best practices, the therapist was following the prescribed treatment modality, but taking into account the life changes Marjorie was experiencing, she was not yet stable.

The therapist sent a new treatment form to the case manager. When the case manager reviewed the treatment form, he contacted the therapist to get a clearer understanding as to why additional sessions were necessary. The case manager had assessed that a total of 16 sessions had been used between the therapist and the psychiatrist. Marjorie had a total of 30 sessions in a calendar year.

The therapist explained that he was concerned about a relapse and that additional sessions would help to solidify the solutions already in place, to strengthen the interpersonal relationships and support systems, and to transition the client to group therapy at a community service agency. The therapist explained that if he could successfully connect Marjorie to group therapy, he believed that she would make the transition successfully and not represent for treatment. Based on the history that the therapist shared with the MCO, the case manager agreed to authorize the additional sessions.

Finally, the therapist completed treatment and submitted a termination summary to the case manager. This case worked well because of the relationship that the therapist had with the MCO. The therapist had partnered with the MCO long enough to have established a practice pattern that was tried and true. The therapist made clinical arguments that were grounded both clinically and within the preferred practice guidelines of the MCO. The case management process generally works best when the case manager has had positive, professional experience with the therapist. Besides the analytical reports on practice patterns, the case manager will look at member satisfaction with the provider, case management history, and the therapist's clinical orientation.

THE FUTURE OF MANAGED CARE

The future of managed care will be based on MCOs ability to manage networks instead of managing cases. Providers will most likely enter the provider panel on the lowest level. The provider will be encouraged, if not required, to attend provider education programs. Once the provider has a certain number of cases and amount of education on which to build, he/she will move to the next level. The MCOs may even establish behavioral measurements to determine success at this stage. Therapists who are unable to achieve success at this level may be dismissed from the provider panel.

The second level will probably offer providers more autonomy. Providers at the second tier will most likely be educated about managing their own cases. Such education would probably include, but not be limited to, benefit packages, designing the course of treatment based on the client's diagnosis and presenting problem, additional emphasis on conducting case coordination with other professionals, and standing orders so that providers can make referrals to ancillary services. These providers will probably have more simplified administrative duties, which may include simplified treatment forms. The therapist will be responsible for submitting treatment forms simply for the MCO to authorize payment.

The highest level will probably be a more autonomous version of the previous level. Assuming technology will eventually be able to support this level, providers will be able to submit their treatment forms directly into a system that could automatically produce an authorization for payment. If such a program is devised, ultimately the MCO case managers will be able to focus on continuous provider education and continuous quality improvement, and to serve as a resource for providers to collaborate on difficult cases.

Interfacing with Other Professionals

Psychiatrists. When the therapist has a client who is on medication, it is important to coordinate his or her care with the psychiatrist so that each party is fully informed. It is essential for the therapist to know what medication the client is on and to become educated about possible side effects and the protocols for stopping medications. This is simply for education purposes; the therapist should never give medication advice.

In turn, the interaction benefits the psychiatrist who will be kept apprised of the client's progress in therapy and who may also find that systemic interventions enhance medication compliance.

Primary Care Physicians. For many MCOs, clients will get a referral to access their mental health benefits through the primary care physician. Even when this is not the case, in general, the primary care physician will be interested in the care of his/her client. It is important to establish a good rapport with the primary care physician. When you communicate the treatment plan, and any behavioral cues that may be pertinent to the general well-being of the client, the primary care physician becomes better prepared to treat the client. In addition, an established relationship with the primary care physician can lead to more referrals.

Home Health Care. There are a number of times that the MCO may call in a home health care agency in order to dispense a client's medication. This is done in conjunction with a psychiatrist. In these situations, it is important to communicate with the home health care agency as well as the psychiatrist. The primary thing to find out for your records is when appointments for the home health care are scheduled. Home health care is usually implemented for clients of high chronicity and limited social support. Therefore, the role of the therapist in these cases is generally psychoeducational.

School Officials/Teachers. Many families come to therapy identifying one of the children as the patient. Many times, the parents will report that a teacher has complained about the child's behavior. At this point, the therapy is focused around a phantom complainant, especially if the parents are not experiencing the same problems at home. It is important to speak with the teacher or school official to obtain that person's understanding of the problem and to let him/her know what your treatment plan is. This sharing of information creates an opportunity for conflicting agendas to be worked out so that treatment can move forward.

Police/Court Officials. Oten a client will initiate clinical care at the request of the legal system. This may mean that the client is not really a customer for change. In these instances, it is important to check with the MCO to see if this course of treatment is covered by the insurance. If it is, it will be necessary to contact the agency making the referral to understand what it is expecting the client to achieve from therapy. This will help you to set a treatment plan and establish a reporting schedule.

Attorneys. Some clients will be represented by attorneys for court cases. The client's attorney may want you to provide a report to be used during a court hearing. Check with the MCO to see if this care will be covered by the insurance. If it is, you need to determine the difference between treatment and evaluation. Once the course is decided, it will be necessary to establish a reporting schedule. It is important that the client be able to contract for change, not just to please the court.

Written Consent for the Release of Information

A release of information is important to the case management process. Required by law in order to disclose confidential information, the written release of information should be completed for any professional caregiver and for any person from whom the therapist needs information or to whom the therapist must give information. The therapist should even have the client fill out a written release of information so that the therapist has permission to contact the MCO case manager and share information that helps the professionals to coordinate the care.

Exhibit 6.1 is an example of a release of information form. As with all legal documents, the therapist should have his/her attorney review the form to be used. This should be a precaution taken by the therapist to make sure that the form is legally sound when used appropriately.

Psychological Testing

Although psychological testing can be done only by psychologists or psychometricians, it is an important topic among therapists who are used to working from a modality of therapy based on testing to determine diagnosis. Recent literature (Bindler & Shapiro, 1995; Ficken, 1995; Hays, 1995; Werthman, 1995; Schlosser, 1995) has attempted to help providers who utilize psychological testing to understand its role in managed behavioral care. In addition, it has attempted to help providers understand the future role that psychological testing may have in managed behavioral care.

It has been argued that psychological testing helps therapists to:

1. Generate a diagnosis.

2. Identify critical problems that require immediate intervention (e.g., suicidality, homicidality, psychosis, substance abuse).

Authorization for the Release of
Confidential Information

Patient Name: _____

Patient Social Security Number: _____

Patient Address: _____

I give my permission for_____(party 1) to
(Name, Address, and Phone Number)

communicate with _____(party 2) verbally or
(Name, Address, and Phone Number)

in writing to coordinate my therapeutic care and share information that will help in this process. The following information should not be shared: _____

_____

_____

_____

This release of information is in effect for ninety (90) days from the date below. I (the patient) understand that I can revoke this authorization at any time simply by informing party 1 or party 2 in writing. My signature below indicates a full understanding of this release.

_____
Patient Signature   Date

_____
Witness   Date

_____
Signature of Guardian   Date
(For patients who are minors)

Exhibit 6.1. Sample release of information form.

3. Flesh out characterlogical factors that can dramatically alter the prognosis and preferred treatment regimen.

4. Provide an index of symptom severity to guide decisions about the necessary level of care (Ficken, 1995). However, in most instances, a thorough clinical assessment can provide the therapist with the same information, and that the information can be gathered in a more timely and cost-efficient manner than with psychological testing. This point is no more apparent than with a client who may be in immediate danger of harming him/herself and/or others. In this case, immediate intervention is required and psychological testing may hinder clinical intervention.

As a general rule, MCOs do not pay for psychological testing unless it is deemed medically necessary, for example, to rule out organicity. One area that has come to the forefront in recent years is testing to determine a diagnosis of Attention Deficit/Hyperactivity Disorder. Werthman (1995) explained that many therapists routinely request psychological testing for this disorder process, and yet, this diagnosis can be determined with a thorough and systemic assessment. In addition, the individual responsible for confirming the diagnosis and determining if medication is indicated would be the child psychiatrist or pediatrician. Therefore, if the therapist feels that the diagnosis is even questionable, he or she should refer the client to the psychiatrist and continue treatment focused on family intervention and behavioral modification.

But psychological testing is not dead. In the future, the focus of testing will be for outcome studies (Ficken, 1995). Outcome assessment tools will have to be developed to serve the needs of therapists and MCOs to show the efficacy of the therapeutic interventions. The goal will be for the outcome assessments to be integrated into the treatment process so that information is gathered immediately.

Finally, therapists must remember that they need to work *with* the MCOs and not against them. As the world of managed behavioral care changes, the therapist needs to be willing to change as well. Therapists will hurt themselves only by trying to hold on to the old ways. Changes need not be a negative thing; they should be viewed as opportunities to challenge therapists to find better, more efficient, and more systemic ways of working. In the long run, this will benefit the professional, the MCO, and most important, the client/client family.

7

A Pragmatic View of Case Management

This chapter presents two case examples in which case management was performed and others in which it was not. From these examples, therapists will be able to clearly see how appropriate case management pays off, not only for the client/family, but for the therapist as well. The following cases were chosen through a retrospective review of MCO cases. The names have been changed to assure confidentiality.

THE "T" FAMILY

The T family entered counseling identifying their 8-year-old daughter as the patient. The therapist began by getting a clear

119

assessment of the problem. Brenda was the biological daughter of Mrs. T. Both Mrs. T's sister and Brenda were living with her when she married Mr. T. Upon presentation, Mr. and Mrs. T had a 4-year-old child, as well as Brenda, and Mrs. T's sister, who had multiple sclerosis, living in their home.

When the family presented for therapy, they stated that Brenda was "a problem child because she was hard to manage and dangerously violent." The therapist immediately felt that more information was needed. Upon obtaining releases of information to speak to Brenda's teachers and pediatrician, the therapist found out that Brenda was enrolled in classes for children with unique learning needs and that it was suspected that Brenda had a pervasive learning disorder. The therapist coordinated through the managed behavioral health care company and through the HMO for Brenda to have a psychiatric evaluation and a neurological examination.

The therapist coordinated this for a number of reasons. For one, the therapist was faced with parents who kept requesting to drop Brenda off for individual therapy and who wanted inpatient hospitalization to "fix" her. It was the hope of the therapist to obtain an accurate diagnosis so that the parents could be educated about the concept that Brenda's "problem" was an "unfixable" problem that would have lasting impact. This would offer an opportunity to teach the parents to understand the fact that they would need to learn how to handle, problem solve, and educate Brenda as she developed.

In addition, a thorough evaluation could provide feedback to the school system so it could readdress Brenda's program needs. By coordinating the information from all professionals involved, the therapist could assure that she put herself in a win–win situation. If the assessment showed that there was not a pervasive developmental problem, then an appropriate therapeutic treatment plan could be established in order to find solutions for the family that might include but not be limited to: family therapy, medication management, a social skills group, and a parenting therapy group. If the assessment showed that there was a pervasive developmental disorder, then the therapist could assist with refocusing the school program, and helping Mr. and Mrs. T to understand Brenda's limitations and to learn different ways to work with Brenda than they would with their younger daughter.

In this case, Brenda's comprehensive evaluation showed that she did have an organic deficiency, which was irreparable. This information was very hard for Mr. and Mrs. T to accept. At first, they fought for inpatient hospitalization in order to get Brenda "fixed." They went through their employer group to add pressure on the therapist to "fix" Brenda. They were also resistant to attending multiple sessions at multiple offices. The therapist explained that Brenda was Mr. and Mrs. T's child and therefore they owned the responsibility for Brenda's treatment.

Mr. and Mrs. T finally caught on to the process and engaged in treatment. Their involvement led them to a new understanding of Brenda's problem and they learned new ways of coping. In addition to this, the case management aided in finding community resources, respite programs, and new schooling. This provided great help to Mr. and Mrs. T, as well as to Brenda. Once therapy ended, Mr. and Mrs. T did not represent in chaotic or crisis-oriented ways.

THE "B" FAMILY

The B family was introduced to the MCO when the 16-year-old son presented for inpatient treatment. John was experi-

encing his first psychotic break. He was religiously preoccu-
pied; would not speak, except for prayer; and sat on his bed
rocking to and fro all day while he hid behind his long hair.
John's older brother had been hospitalized with the same diagnosis, and the mother had received the same diagnosis but
had refused treatment. John experienced great difficulty clear-
ing from his psychosis and spent more than 30 days in a psychiatric hospital with various medication trials until the
appropriate combination was found.

When John was discharged from the hospital, he was connected with a family therapist and a psychiatrist. The family
therapist saw the entire family for the first two sessions. He
made many suggestions. He requested that the parents look
for unique-needs schooling, that they get connected to
a parenting group, and that John get connected to a family
service board so that he could get funding for vocational
rehabilitation.

Each week the therapist would ask the family if they had
followed through and then would go through all the reasons
why they had not, trying to get them motivated. When they
saw the psychiatrist, the family would report that they did
not understand the therapist's approach and could not understand why the therapist was giving them so many telephone numbers. Because the therapist did not coordinate/
communicate with the psychiatrist, this information was never
retrieved. The family soon dropped out of therapy. Although
John showed some improvement through the aid of psycho-
pharmacology, he did not learn new coping strategies or get
the special educational services that were appropriate. John
gradually started to decompensate as the craziness remained
around him, and he had no way of appropriately handling it.
John did represent for hospitalization. Because he had no
inpatient benefits left for the calendar year, he was remanded
to a community mental health agency.

The above cases exemplify how good case management

provides the best possible clinical services to the client. In the first case, the therapist was faced with a family that initially was not invested in extended services because they did not understand the real problem. As the therapist followed through with comprehensive case management, she provided the family with new information that helped the family to comprehend the problem in a new way. In addition, the case management process gave information to the therapist as to how to develop the treatment plan, which in turn allowed the therapy to be more meaningful. By utilizing the resources that were available, the therapist worked from the most informed position possible.

In the second case, the therapist did not facilitate the case management. Instead, he tried to put the ownership on a client family that was unable to do the necessary networking on their own. By not speaking to the psychiatrist, the therapist missed an opportunity to get valuable feedback. It is impossible to be certain, but had the appropriate case management been in place, John might have been able to avoid another hospitalization.

8

Remember This

INTRODUCTION

Given that all of this information can be somewhat confusing to the provider who is being exposed to managed care for the first time, this chapter looks at some of the most important things to remember. It is essential to become comfortable with the fact of a changing environment, as the most stable thing about managed care is that it is ever-changing. The therapist should be successful in a managed care environment if he/she holds on to the following skills.

125

Skills for Success

Therapy needs to be focused primarily on the here and now. Therapy plans that focus on the client's present needs are best accepted by MCOs. This is not to suggest that therapy is merely a patch. Brief systemic therapies that stay focused on finding solutions to present problems have proved to be useful in helping clients to discover coping strategies that they can apply to a variety of other problems. MCOs are looking for the most effective way to work with clients while remaining within the limited number of sessions that the client has available.

Problems need to be defined behaviorally, and treatment plans must clearly state how solutions will be achieved. When problems are defined behaviorally, it is easy to set clearly measurable goals. This helps the client and the therapist measure the client's success. In addition to these obvious advantages, it also helps the MCO to define the medical necessity for a given case.

Treatment plans must state how both the client and the therapist will know solutions have been established and that it is time to terminate therapy. This is a common error on the part of the therapist. Often the termination of therapy is not discussed from the onset. Discharge planning should be done from the first session. This lets the client understand that there will be an end to the therapy and helps the client to define that end.

The average length of treatment for adjustment disorder and V-Code diagnoses is 8 to 10 sessions. When you can state with confidence that you are hitting this benchmark and show that your clients are satisfied with the services they received, you will be viewed as a therapist who has good potential for success in the managed care environment.

Stay open to feedback and change. Since the provider wants to build a partnership with MCOs, the provider needs to be open to feedback. In addition, being open to feedback will keep the provider aligned with the constant changes of the managed care world.

Join with the companies that fit with your professional and personal ethics. Panelship with MCOs that match your professional and personal ethics, will mean less potential difficulty partnering with the MCO. When your ethics are not in sync with the business and/or clinical practices of an MCO, you will find yourself in a constant battle. Do not go into the relationship believing that you will change the MCO.

Good case management skills. Coordinating the care of your client is a valuable tool that will help the client get more out of the therapeutic process. There are a number of professionals and paraprofessionals with whom the provider will need to coordinate:

> *Psychiatrists.* Systemic intervention usually helps with medication compliance. Obtain medication information and side effects. Ask the psychiatrist what information he/she wants from you and set up a reporting process.

> *Primary Care Physicians.* Inform the primary care physician that the client is in treatment and provide information about the treatment plan. Inform the primary care physician of any changes in treatment, including the termination of the therapeutic process. In addition, find out if the client is on medication(s) and coordinate treatment needs.

Home Health Care. If the client is receiving home health care, find out who prescribes the medications, the schedule for home health care visits, and the extent of treatment that the agency will perform. By coordinating this care, the therapist can inventory the services provided and ensure that services will not be duplicated or be counterproductive.

School Officials/Teachers. By bringing these professionals' voices into the treatment, the therapist starts to address the complaints that they may have initiated. Even in cases where these professionals are not the chief complainants, including them in the treatment helps build in success for the client/family.

Court Officials/Attorneys. As in the above, it is important to understand the needs of all involved. Often the client is coming to therapy at the suggestion of some one else. When involved in the court system, the client usually follows the agenda of the system and often without a clear understanding of the reasons. The therapist can facilitate treatment by gathering the information from the court officials.

Available appointment times. Find out if the MCOs have access standards. If so, make sure that your schedule and case load can support the MCO's access standards. If at any time you cannot take on new cases, request that the MCO stop sending you referrals until your case load opens up.

Ask questions about various benefits packages. Ask the MCOs to educate you regarding the various benefit packages that they manage. Remember that within a company there may be different benefit packages.

Treatment plan cheat sheet. Always make sure that the

following information is included in your initial treatment plan: client's name, client and subscriber's Social Security numbers, date of assessment, presenting problem, psychosocial information, mental status examination, diagnosis, treatment goals, and action plan.

Treatment summary cheat sheet. The following information should be included in a treatment summary: client's name and Social Security number, updated diagnosis, estimated number of sessions to complete treatment, changes in symptoms, response to treatment, revisions to treatment plan, and updated treatment plan.

Organize MCO requirements. Whether it be different colored files, cheat sheets, or separate ledgers in each file, the therapist needs to understand the policies and procedures of each MCO. It is also essential to keep straight the reporting schedule and documentation required for each MCO.

Do not triangulate the client and MCO. As a therapist, you need to be reminded that you are an extended representative of the MCO. As such, when you negotiate the appropriate level of care with the MCO, the MCO will expect you to report these decisions back to the client as a mutual decision. For example, it may be therapeutically appropriate for a client who is experiencing depression to see a psychiatrist for a medication evaluation when the depressive symptoms do not subside. If the case manager asks you to help facilitate this request with the client, it will be more advantageous to the client if you present this as a joint decision on the part of you and the MCO. Do not present it as "the MCO wants you to or told you to...." It may need to be addressed as a therapeutic issue if the client does not understand the decision.

CONCLUSION

There are many opportunities for therapists with MCOs. The relationships can be positive and plentiful. As with all relationships, there are often rough times. Until now, MCOs and therapists have been courting one another. Many of the initial relationships have not lasted. However, the courting phase has progressed to an engagement for many therapists—those who remained flexible and were willing to ride through the rough times. Now, the industry is on the verge of a true marriage. Family therapists are best aligned for such a marriage. The most progressive MCOs will learn to learn from their providers to create feedback loops that will streamline the work flows of case management processes, to be cost-effective, and most importantly, to provide clients with the highest quality of care possible.

Glossary

Administrative Services Only (ASO). A self-funded benefit approach where claims are administered through a purely administrative arrangement with the employer.

Authorization. Approval from managed care organization that provides parameters for covered care.

Calendar Year Benefit. A benefit period that runs from January 1 to December 31 of each year.

Carve Out. Separating out a specific piece of a benefit program to contract separately, providing greater expertise or better access.

Case Management. The process by which the clinical care is organized and coordinated among all involved professionals and the managed care organization.

Client. An MCO member accessing services.

Copayment. The payments for a covered expense that are shared by the insurance company and the insured. A copay is usually a fixed dollar amount and refers to the client's liability.

Employee Assistance Program (EAP). Assessment and referral program pre-purchased by employer.

Employer. The insurance subscriber's place of work.

Exclusive Provider Organization (EPO). A form of preferred provider organization (PPO) that is rigidly structured to the point of resembling an HMO. Employees must go only to the providers who contract with the plan. No payment is made for treatment by any other provider.

Fee for Service. Payment is made on the basis of each incident of service.

Health Maintenance Organization (HMO). Fixed fee covers all services needed by members; controls which provider supplies services.

Indemnity. Pays third-party payment to any provider.

Managed Care Organization (MCO). Sell utilization review services to HMOs, PPOs, insurers, and companies to gate-keep and review access to mental health services. They establish contractual agreements with providers through an application process. Sometimes they act as providers as well.

Managed Indemnity. Requires precertification for surgical procedures only.

Point of Service (POS). An HMO-like product where the employee chooses a network provider when services are needed; out-of-network services are covered at reduced benefits.

Preauthorization. Authorization for payment that occurs prior to the services being rendered.

Preferred Provider Organization (PPO). This program channels patients to providers who have contracted discount fees by giving the members a list of these providers to choose from.

Release of Information. A written authorization that gives the therapist permission to speak with and coordinate care with other professionals and the managed care organization. In addition, a release of information should be prepared if the client wants information released to anyone.

Termination Summary. A statement produced by the therapist that summarizes the course of treatment and the reason for case closure.

Treatment Plan. A written or oral plan of action for the course of therapy produced by the therapist and shared with the client. The treatment plan should outline the treatment goals and the action plans to meet the stated goals.

Treatment Update. A written or oral statement produced by the therapist that states where the therapy started, where the therapy is currently, and what goals still need to be achieved in order to terminate therapy. This statement is shared with the MCO case manager so that continued authorization can be provided.

Utilization Review (UR). The evaluation of the necessity, appropriateness, and efficiency of all services, procedures, and resources. Review items include treatment plan, intensity and level of care, treatment modality, and setting.

References

Bateson, G., Jackson, D. D., Haley, J., & Weakland, J. (1956). Toward a theory of schizophrenia. *Behavioral Science, 1,* 251–264.

Bindler, P. R. & Shapiro, R. (1995). Psychological testing in brief Psychotherapy. *Behavioral Health Management, September/October,* 18–20.

de Shazer, S. (1985). *Keys to solutions in brief therapy.* New York: Norton.

de Shazer, S., Berg, I. K., Lipchick, E., Nunnaly, E., Molnar, A., Gingerich, W., & Weiner-Davis, M. (1986). Brief therapy: Focused solution development. *Family Process, 25,* 207–222.

Ficken J. (1995). New directions for psychological testing: How psychological testing can be reoriented to become managed care friendly. *Behavioral Health Management, September/October,* 12–14.

Fisch, R., Weakland, J. H., & Segal, L. (1982). *The tactics of change: Doing therapy briefly.* San Francisco: Jossey-Bass.

Garfield, S., & Bergin, A. (Eds.). (1978). *Handbook of psychotherapy and behavior change* (2nd ed.). New York: Wiley.

Giles, T. R. (Ed.). (1993). *Handbook of effective psycho-therapy*. New York: Plenum Press.

Goldberg, J. F., & Harrow, M. (1994). Kindling in bipolar disorders: A longitudinal follow-up study. *Society of Biological Psychiatry, 35,* 70–72.

Haley, J. (1976). *Problem-solving therapy*. San Francisco: Jossey-Bass.

Haley, J. (1980). *Leaving home*. New York: McGraw-Hill.

Haley, J. (Ed.). (1985). *Conversations with Milton H. Erickson: Vol. 2. Changing individuals*. New York: Triangle Press.

Hays, L. W. (1995). Relating psychological testing to prognosis and outcomes. *Behavioral Health Management, September/October,* 21–25.

Koss, M. P. (1979). Length of psychotherapy for clients seen in private practice. *Journal of Consulting and Clinical Psychology, 47,* 210–212.

Madanes, C. (1980). Protection, paradox, and pretending. *Family Process, 19,* 73–85.

Madanes, C. (1981). *Strategic family therapy*. San Francisco: Jossey-Bass.

Madanes, C., & Haley, J. (1977). Dimensions of family therapy. *Journal of Nervous and Mental Disease, 165,* 88–98.

Marek, L. I., Sandifer, D. M., Beach, A., Coward, R. L., & Protinsky, H. O. (1994). Supervision without the problem: A model of solution-focused supervision. *Journal of Family Psychotherapy, 5,* 57–64.

Minuchin, S. (1974). *Families and family therapy*. Cambridge, Mass. Harvard University Press.

Minuchin, S., & Fishman, H. C. (1981). *Family therapy techniques*. Cambridge, Mass. Harvard University Press.

O'Hanlon, W. H., & Weiner-Davis, M. (1989). *In search of solutions: A new direction in psychotherapy*. New York: Norton.

Penn. (1982). Circular questioning. *Family Process, 21*(3), 267–280.

Piercy, F. P., & Sprenkle, D. H. (1986). *Family therapy sourcebook.* New York: Guilford.

Poynter, W. L. (1994). *The preferred provider's handbook: Building a successful private therapy practice in the managed care marketplace.* New York: Brunner/Mazel.

Rosen, S. (1982). *My voice will go with you: The teaching tales of Milton H. Erickson, M.D.* New York: Norton.

Schlosser, B. (1995). Psychological testing: Past and future. *Behavioral Health Management, September/October,* 8–10.

Selekman, M. D., & Todd, T. C. (1995). Co-creating a context for change in the supervisory system: The solution-focused supervision model. *Journal of Systemic Therapies, 49*(3), 21–33.

Selvini Palazzoli, M., Boscolo, G., Cecchin, G., & Prata, G. (1980). Hypothesizing—circularity—neutrality: Three guidelines for the conductor of family interviews. *Family Process, 19,* 3–12.

Selvini Palazzoli, M., Boscolo, G., Cecchin, G., & Prata, G. (1978). *Paradox and counterparadox.* New York: Jason Aronson.

Shilts, I.., & Gordon, A. (1993). Simplifying the miracle. *Family Therapy Case Studies, 7*(2), 53–59.

Thomas, F. N. (1994). Solution-oriented supervision: The coaxing of expertise. *The Family Journal, 2,* 11–18.

Todd, T. C., & Selekman, M. D. (1991). Beyond structural-strategic family therapy. In T. C. Todd & M. D. Selekman (Eds.), *Family therapy approaches with adolescent substance abusers.* Needham Heights, Mass. Allyn & Bacon.

Tomm, C. (1984). One perspective on the Milan systemic approach: Part II. Description of session format, interviewing style and intervention. *Journal of Marital and Family Therapy, 10,* 253-271.

Watzlawick, P., Weakland, J., & Fisch, R. (1974). *Change: Principles of problem formation and problem resolution.* New York: Norton.

Welchler, J. L. (1990). Solution-oriented supervision. *Family Therapy, 17,* 129–138.

Werthman, M. J. (1995). A managed care approach to psychological testing: Far from discounting psychological testing entirely, managed care can enhance its therapeutic usefulness. *Behavioral Health Management, September/October,* 15–17.

Name Index

Subject Index

A

Administrative information, Managed Care Organization (MCO), 6–7

Appointment times, case management and, 128

Attention-deficit/hyperactivity disorder (ADHD), 67, 70, 116

Attorneys, case management and, 113, 128

B

Behavioral model
managed care and, 126
Mental Research Institute (MRI) approach, 38–44

Benefit package, case management and, 128

Brief Family Therapy Center (BFTC), solution-focused approach, 45–56

Brief therapy modalities, 37–85
MCO and, 37
Mental Research Institute (MRI), 38–44
Milan approach, 77–85
skills required, 126–129
solution-focused approach, 45–56
strategic approach, 57–68
structural approach, 68–77

C

Case management, 87–123
case example, 88–93
communication problems, 95–105
financial focus, 105–107
future trends, 110–117
consent forms, 113–114, 115
professional interfaces, 111–113, 127–128
psychological testing, 114, 116–117
interface protocol, 94
language and, 93–94
overview, 87–88
as partnership, 107–110
pragmatic view of, case examples, 119–123
professionalism, 94
skills required, 127–128
structural approach and, 74–77